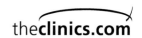

HEMATOLOGY/ ONCOLOGY CLINICS OF NORTH AMERICA

Cancer Survivorship

GUEST EDITORS
Lois B. Travis, MD, ScD
and Joachim Yahalom, MD

April 2008 • Volume 22 • Number 2

SAUNDERS

An Imprint of Elsevier, Inc.
PHILADELPHIA   LONDON   TORONTO   MONTREAL   SYDNEY   TOKYO

W.B. SAUNDERS COMPANY
A Division of Elsevier Inc.

Elsevier Inc. • 1600 John F. Kennedy Boulevard • Suite 1800 • Philadelphia, Pennsylvania 19103-2899

http://www.hemonc.theclinics.com

HEMATOLOGY/ONCOLOGY CLINICS
OF NORTH AMERICA   Volume 22, Number 2
April 2008   ISSN 0889-8588
Editor: Kerry Holland   ISBN-13: 978-1-4160-5843-4
                               ISBN-10: 1-4160-5843-5

Reprints: For copies of 100 or more, of articles in this publication, please contact the Commercial Reprints Department, Elsevier Inc., 360 Park Avenue South, New York, New York 10010-1710. Tel. (212) 633-3813; Fax: (212) 462-1935; E-mail: reprints@elsevier.com.

The ideas and opinions expressed in *Hematology/Oncology Clinics of North America* do not necessarily reflect those of the Publisher. The Publisher does not assume any responsibility for any injury and/or damage to persons or property arising out of or related to any use of the material contained in this periodical. The reader is advised to check the appropriate medical literature and the product information currently provided by the manufacturer of each drug to be administered to verify the dosage, the method and duration of administration, or contraindications. It is the responsibility of the treating physician or other health care professional, relying on independent experience and knowledge of the patient, to determine drug dosages and the best treatment of the patient. Mention of any product in this issue should not be construed as endorsement by the contributors, editors, or the Publisher of the product or manufacturers' claims.

Hematology/Oncology Clinics (ISSN 0889-8588) is published bimonthly by Elsevier Inc., 360 Park Avenue South, New York, NY 10010-1710. Months of issue are February, April, June, August, October, and December. Business and Editorial Offices: 1600 John F. Kennedy Blvd., Suite 1800, Philadelphia, PA 19103-2899. Customer Service Office: 6277 Sea Harbor Drive, Orlando, FL 32887-4800. Periodicals postage paid at New York, NY and additional mailing offices. Subscription prices are $262.00 per year (US individuals), $392.00 per year (US institutions), $131.00 per year (US students), $297.00 per year (Canadian individuals), $470.00 per year (Canadian institutions), $166.00 per year (Canadian students), $332.00 per year (international individuals), $470.00 per year (international institutions), $166.00 per year (international students). International air speed delivery is included in all *Clinics* subscription prices. All prices are subject to change without notice. **POSTMASTER:** Send address changes to *Hematology/Oncology Clinics of North America*, Elsevier Periodicals Customer Service, 6277 Sea Harbor Drive, Orlando, FL 32887-4800. Customer Service: 1-800-654-2452 (US). From outside the United States, call 1-407-563-6020. Fax: 1-407-363-9661. E-mail: JournalsCustomerService-usa@elsevier.com.

Hematology/Oncology Clinics of North America is covered in *Index Medicus, EMBASE/Excerpta Medica,* and *BIOSIS.*

Printed in the United States of America.

Cancer Survivorship

GUEST EDITORS

LOIS B. TRAVIS, MD, ScD, Senior Investigator (Adjunct), Division of Cancer Epidemiology and Genetics, National Cancer Institute, Department of Health and Human Services, National Institutes of Health, Bethesda, Maryland

JOACHIM YAHALOM, MD, Attending and Member, Department of Radiation Oncology, Memorial Sloan-Kettering Cancer Center; Professor of Radiation Oncology, Weill Medical College of Cornell University, New York, New York

CONTRIBUTORS

JAMES M. ALLAN, DPhil, Northern Institute for Cancer Research, Medical School, Newcastle University, Newcastle upon Tyne, United Kingdom

KEITH M. BELLIZZI, PhD, MPH, Program Director, Office of Cancer Survivorship, Division of Cancer Control and Population Sciences, National Cancer Institute, Department of Health and Human Services, National Institutes of Health, Bethesda, Maryland

BARRIE CASSILETH, MS, PhD, Laurance S. Rockefeller Chair in Integrative Medicine; and Chief, Integrative Medicine Service, Memorial Sloan-Kettering Cancer Center, New York, New York

ALV A. DAHL, MD, PhD, Professor, Department of Clinical Cancer Research, Norwegian Radium Hospital, Rikshospitalet University Hospital, Montebello; Faculty Division, The Norwegian Radium Hospital, University of Oslo, Oslo, Norway

WENDY DEMARK-WAHNEFRIED, PhD, RD, Professor of Behavioral Science, Department of Behavioral Science, The University of Texas–MD Anderson Cancer Center, Houston, Texas

SOPHIE D. FOSSÅ, MD, PhD, Professor, Department of Clinical Cancer Research, Norwegian Radium Hospital, Rikshospitalet University Hospital, Montebello; Faculty Division, The Norwegian Radium Hospital, University of Oslo, Oslo, Norway

MARY GOSPODAROWICZ, MD, FRCPC, FRCR (Hon), Professor and Chair, Department of Radiation Oncology, University of Toronto; Medical Director, Cancer Program, Princess Margaret Hospital, Toronto, Ontario, Canada

JYOTHIRMAI GUBILI, MS, Assistant Editor, Integrative Medicine Service, Memorial Sloan-Kettering Cancer Center, New York, New York

DAVID C. HODGSON, MD, MPH, Associate Professor, Department of Radiation Oncology, University of Toronto, Princess Margaret Hospital, Toronto, Canada

SANDRA J. HORNING MD, Professor of Medicine, Stanford University, Stanford, California

MELISSA M. HUDSON, MD, Professor, Department of Pediatrics, LeBonheur Children's Medical Center, University of Tennessee College of Medicine; Member, Department of Oncology; and Director, Division of Cancer Survivorship, St. Jude Children's Research Hospital, Memphis, Tennessee

LEE W. JONES, PhD, Assistant Research Professor of Surgery, Department of Surgery, Duke University Medical Center, Durham, North Carolina

SUSAN LEIGH, BSN, RN, Cancer Survivorship Consultant and Founding Member, National Coalition for Cancer Survivorship, Tucson, Arizona

ANDREA K. NG, MD, MPH, Associate Professor of Radiation Oncology, Department of Radiation Oncology, Dana-Farber Cancer Institute, Brigham and Women's Hospital, Harvard Medical School, Boston, Massachusetts

CAROL S. PORTLOCK, MD, Department of Medicine, Memorial Sloan-Kettering Cancer Center, New York, New York

JULIA H. ROWLAND, PhD, Director, Office of Cancer Survivorship, Division of Cancer Control and Population Sciences, National Cancer Institute, Department of Health and Human Services, National Institutes of Health, Bethesda, Maryland

LOIS B. TRAVIS, MD, ScD, Senior Investigator (Adjunct), Division of Cancer Epidemiology and Genetics, National Cancer Institute, Department of Health and Human Services, National Institutes of Health, Bethesda, Maryland

KATHLEEN WESA, MD, Assistant Attending Physician, Integrative Medicine Service, Memorial Sloan-Kettering Cancer Center, New York, New York

JOACHIM YAHALOM, MD, Attending and Member, Department of Radiation Oncology, Memorial Sloan-Kettering Cancer Center; Professor of Radiation Oncology, Weill Medical College of Cornell University, New York, New York

Cancer Survivorship

who are at increased risk for a variety of health problems resulting from their cancer or its treatment. Risk-based survivor care is recommended for all survivors. To optimize risk-based survivor care, several groups have organized health screening guidelines based on evidence from the literature linking specific therapeutic interventions with late treatment complications. This article addresses the scope of long-term health effects after pediatric cancer, the challenges in coordinating long-term survivor care, and health screening guideline resources available to facilitate survivor care.

Hodgkin lymphoma (HL) is a disease that typically strikes children and young adults, with more than 80% of those affected being cured. Consequently, HL survivors can live for decades with the persistent and late-emerging effects of the disease and its treatment. The focus of this article is the long-term medical management of HL survivors, specifically those who are 5 years or more off therapy without evidence of relapse, when the focus of follow-up care shifts from detecting relapse to minimizing the morbidity associated with the late effects of treatment.

Over the past 30 years, testicular tumors have become the paradigm for a curable adult cancer. Numerous factors have contributed to this success, including the introduction of newer treatment approaches, such as cisplatin-based combination chemotherapy and curative retroperitoneal lymph node dissection. Moreover, the last three decades have witnessed the evolution of newer diagnostic methods, improvements in staging, the evaluation of patient response, and the monitoring of relapse. These treatment successes have been accompanied by the emergence of the late effects of testicular cancer and its treatment, including second primary cancers, cardiovascular sequelae, the metabolic syndrome, gonadal toxicity, neurotoxicity, and pulmonary sequelae. An overview of these late effects and recommendations for patient follow-up are presented in this article.

Constitutional (hereditary) genetic variation and somatic genetic alterations acquired during transformation to the neoplastic phenotype are both critical determinants of cancer outcome, and can ultimately have a significant effect on cancer survivorship. This article discusses the role of constitutional and somatic genetics in determining outcome and survivorship following a diagnosis of cancer using illustrative examples primarily from the hematologic malignancies.

Andrea K. Ng and Lois B. Travis

Substantial improvements in the past few decades in cancer detection and supportive care along with advances in therapy have led to growing numbers of cancer survivors. In view of the prolongation of survival in increasing numbers of patients, identification and quantification of the late effects of cancer and its therapy have become critical. One of the most serious events experienced by cancer survivors is the diagnosis of a new cancer. The number of patients who have second or higher-order cancers is increasing, and solid tumors are a leading cause of mortality among several populations of long-term survivors, including patients who have Hodgkin lymphoma. The focus of this article is treatment-associated malignancies in survivors of selected adult cancers.

Sophie D. Fosså and Alv A. Dahl

Post-treatment fertility and sexuality are important issues to be considered before treatment starts in young adult patients who have cancer. Most male cancer survivors who have malignancies typical for young adulthood preserve the potential to father a child. Fertility remains decreased in comparable females treated for cancer in reproductive years. Postdiagnosis sexual life is affected, more so in females than in males, and was found to be strongly associated with emotional aspects of partnership. Communication about fertility and sexuality must become an integrated part of cancer survivors' follow-up.

Joachim Yahalom and Carol S. Portlock

Cardiac complications resulting from chemotherapy and radiation pose a significant risk for morbidity and mortality to the cancer survivor. Cardiac side effects may progress over time and are a concern for patients treated during childhood. Long-term pulmonary complications are relatively infrequent, and acute respiratory effects of drugs (mostly bleomycin) or radiation normally resolve early after therapy. Although most cardiovascular risk statistics and clinical experience are derived from patients treated before 1985, the modern radiation approach that limits the exposure of the heart and reduces the total dose seems to attenuate the previously observed cardiovascular risk. Potential preventive measures for high-risk patients are of increasing interest but remain experimental.

Promoting a Healthy Lifestyle Among Cancer Survivors 319
Wendy Demark-Wahnefried and Lee W. Jones

With improving longevity, the late-occurring adverse effects of cancer and its treatment are becoming increasingly apparent. As in other clinical populations, healthy lifestyle behaviors encompassing weight management, a healthy diet, regular exercise, and smoking cessation have the potential to reduce morbidity and mortality significantly in cancer survivors. This article addresses the strength of evidence for recommendations in areas of weight management, diet, exercise, and smoking cessation; and the current evidence examining the efficacy of various intervention approaches to promote health behavior changes among adult cancer survivors.

Integrative Oncology: Complementary Therapies for Cancer Survivors 343
Kathleen Wesa, Jyothirmai Gubili, and Barrie Cassileth

Cancer survivors experience a wide range of symptoms during and following completion of treatment, and some of these symptoms may persist for years or even decades. While pharmacologic treatments relieve many symptoms, they too may produce difficult side effects. Complementary therapies are noninvasive, inexpensive, and useful in controlling symptoms and improving quality of life, and they may be accessed by patients themselves. Rigorous scientific research has produced evidence that acupuncture, massage therapy, music, and mind-body therapies effectively and safely reduce physical and emotional symptoms. These therapies provide a favorable risk-benefit ratio and permit cancer survivors to help manage their own care.

Cancer Survivorship: Advocacy Organizations and Support Systems 355
Susan Leigh

When oncology evolved into a specialized field of medicine more than four decades ago, the primary goals of most cancer treatment included the extension of patients' life expectancies and the occasional hope for cure. Physicians were seen as the principal and solitary advocate for patients, and information regarding cancer diagnosis, treatment, and side effects was delivered or screened by a doctor. Patient education materials were scarce, formalized support systems were nonexistent, and the future was often difficult to define. Patient advocacy has since expanded to models of self, organizational, and public policy advocacy. This article provides examples of advocacy organizations and support systems that offer guidance to providers and patients throughout the continuum of cancer care and into longer-term survival.

In the last three decades, the number of cancer survivors in the United States has tripled and is growing by 2% each year. In 2004, there were an estimated 10.7 million cancer survivors (representing 3.5% of the United States population) with a concomitant effect on public health. The growing and heterogeneous population of cancer survivors provides important opportunities for clinical and epidemiologic research into cancer biology, long-term treatment effects, prevention, and interventional research. In this article, the authors briefly review the history of the efforts that served to coalesce efforts to champion survivorship research, identify future challenges, and provide a perspective on future recommendations.

FORTHCOMING ISSUES

RECENT ISSUES

THE CLINICS ARE NOW AVAILABLE ONLINE!

Access your subscription at:
http://www.theclinics.com

Preface

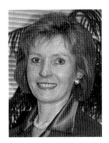 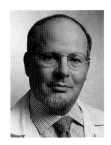

Lois B. Travis, MD, ScD
Joachim Yahalom, MD

Guest Editors

Since 1971, the number of cancer survivors in the United States has tripled, and that number is growing by 2% each year. As of 2005, there were 10.5 million cancer survivors, who comprise 3.5% of the United States population. The burgeoning numbers reflect improvements throughout the cancer continuum, including early detection, supportive care, and therapeutic approaches. This special issue of *Hematology and Oncology Clinics of North America* builds on the considerable momentum that cancer survivorship has gained over the last twenty years (see the article by Drs. Travis and Yahalom). Articles in this issue include "An Overview of Cancer Survivorship in 2008" by Dr. Julia Rowland, who is the current Director of the National Cancer Institute's Office of Cancer Survivorship. New paradigms in the follow-up care of cancer survivors, including initiatives of the American Society of Clinical Oncology (ASCO), are summarized by former ASCO President, Dr. Sandra Horning. Other articles describe the follow-up of survivors of childhood cancer (see the article by Dr. Hudson), testicular cancer (see the article by Dr. Gospodarowicz), and Hodgkin lymphoma (see the article by Dr. Hodgson). Given that many of these patients are cured, a considerable body of literature describing late effects has emerged. Selected sequelae of cancer treatment, including second primary cancers (discussed by Drs. Ng and Travis), cardio-pulmonary toxicity (discussed by Drs. Yahalom and Portlock), and infertility and sexual dysfunction (discussed by Dr. Fossa) also are delineated in this issue. A separate article, written by Dr. Allan, is devoted to the evolving field of the molecular genetics of cancer survivorship. Other articles discuss the promotion of healthy lifestyles among cancer survivors (see the article by Dr. Demark-Wahnefried)

0889-8588/08/$ – see front matter
doi:10.1016/j.hoc.2008.02.001

and the existence of advocacy organizations and support systems (see the article by Dr. Leigh).

Despite the considerable momentum that the topic of cancer survivorship has gained in the last few decades, an enormous amount of work remains to be done to achieve success throughout the cancer trajectory, which is detailed in the enclosed articles. This special edition of *Hematology and Oncology Clinics of North America,* with its broad spectrum of articles devoted to cancer survivorship, will provide an important update to survivors, clinicians, and researchers. Moreover, this issue will continue to provide the field with the attention that it so importantly deserves.

Lois B. Travis, MD, ScD
Division of Cancer Epidemiology and Genetics
National Cancer Institute
Department of Health and Human Services
National Institutes of Health
Bethesda, MD, USA

E-mail address: travis1122@optonline.net

Joachim Yahalom, MD
Department of Radiation Oncology
Memorial Sloan-Kettering Cancer Center
1275 York Avenue
New York, NY 10021, USA

E-mail address: yahalomj@mskcc.org

Cancer Survivors and Survivorship Research: A Reflection on Today's Successes and Tomorrow's Challenges

Julia H. Rowland, PhD*, Keith M. Bellizzi, PhD, MPH

Office of Cancer Survivorship, Division of Cancer Control and Population Sciences, National Cancer Institute, Department of Health and Human Services, National Institutes of Health, 6116 Executive Boulevard, Suite 404, MSC 8336, Bethesda, MD 20892, USA

CANCER SURVIVORSHIP: COMING OF AGE

The past several years have seen an unprecedented increase in the attention being paid to the topic of cancer survivorship. This increase is reflected in the publication of five major reports addressing the status of the research and care of those living with cancer. These include two volumes produced by the Institute of Medicine, *Childhood Cancer Survivorship: Improving Care and Quality of Life* [1], which appeared in August 2003, and *From Cancer Patient to Cancer Survivor: Lost in Transition* [2], released November 2005; a report published in April 2004 by the Centers for Disease Control and Prevention (CDC) and the Lance Armstrong Foundation, *A National Action Plan for Cancer Survivorship to Advance Public Health Strategies* [3]; and two reports from the President's Cancer Panel, *Living Beyond Cancer: Finding a New Balance* [4], released June 2004 with recommendations for consideration, and a follow-up report delivered June 2006, *Assessing Progress, Advancing Change* [5]. Major noncancer and cancer scientific journals, including the *Journal of Pediatric Psychology*, *American Journal of Nursing*, and the *Journal of Clinical Oncology*, have devoted special issues to this aspect of the cancer control continuum [6–8], new texts have appeared summarizing our accomplishments in the field of survivorship research and promoting evidence-based care [9,10], and there is even a new scientific journal to feature this burgeoning area of science [11]. Survivors' stories now routinely appear in diverse news media and print and the yellow "LiveStrong" wrist bands, symbolic of the new face of cancer survivorship so brilliantly championed by Lance Armstrong, can be seen everywhere. Why all the attention? The answer is in the numbers.

In December 1971 when President Nixon signed into law the National Cancer Act and launched what would quickly become referred to as the war on cancer, there were an estimated 3 million cancer survivors in the United States. In this earlier period, the prospect for individuals diagnosed with cancer was bleak.

*Corresponding author. E-mail address: rowlandj@mail.nih.gov (J.H. Rowland).

0889-8588/08/$ – see front matter
doi:10.1016/j.hoc.2008.01.008

Published by Elsevier Inc.
hemonc.theclinics.com

Relatively few treatment options were available; of those that existed, many had serious side effects that were often poorly controlled, and few of these treatments were successful in curing or controlling the illness. It would not be until the late 1970s that 5-year survival rates for all cancers combined would pass the 50% mark. Further, in this earlier period limited resources existed to support patients and their families faced with cancer, and the social stigma attached to the disease meant that one rarely heard cancer discussed either in public or in private. An idea of how grim the outlook was is reflected in the finding that more than 90% of United States physicians during that earlier period said they would not tell their cancer patients their diagnosis [12]. Most psychosocial efforts were geared toward helping patients die of their disease, not live with it, and supporting their family members through the loss of a loved one. Arguably it was these latter individuals who were the cancer survivors during this earlier era.

Today, the picture is dramatically different. As we race into the new millennium, armed with information about the human genome, our ability to cure and control the many diseases termed "cancer" is beginning to make the dream of yesterday become the reality of the present. A major testament to the many successes that have been achieved in the war on cancer is the growing population of survivors. Cancer prevalence figures for the United States have been growing at a rate of approximately 3% per year, and are rapidly approaching 11 million [13], representing approximately 3.6% of the population (Fig. 1). Several factors have contributed to this trend. These include improvements in and broader use of newer cancer screening technologies, more effective–often multimodal and multi-agent combination–therapies, greater application of adjuvant treatments, better supportive care, and growing attention to surveillance once treatment ends.

All of these advances, however, have resulted in treatments being more complex and the decisions regarding these often complicated, and a greater need for help negotiating the lengthy cancer experience that for many will last years or even a lifetime. It has also made us begin to attend to the pressing question: At what cost to individuals, families, and society, do we seek to cure or, as is the case for growing numbers, control these diseases we call cancer? The growing population of cancer survivors and the increasingly vocal advocacy of many of its members serve as reminders that we have an obligation to look beyond the search for a cure and to address the needs of, and provide hope for a valued future to, those living with and beyond a cancer diagnosis. This demand lent urgency to and continues to fuel the development of the still-young field of cancer survivorship research.

In the sections that follow, we describe the characteristics of today's cancer survivors, project the profile of tomorrow's survivors, describe the current field of survivorship research and what it is telling us, and outline some of the major challenges facing cancer survivorship research for the future.

A PROFILE OF TODAY'S SURVIVORS

In 2004, the year for which we have the most current data, it is estimated that the number of cancer survivors in the United States was 10.8 million [14],

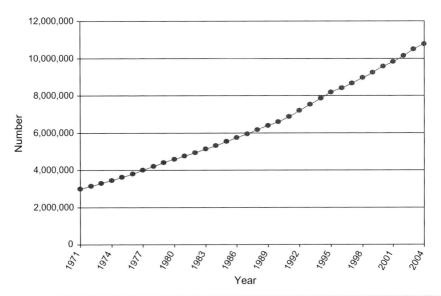

Fig. 1. Estimated number of cancer survivors in the United States from 1971 to 2004. (*From* National Cancer Institute. Cancer control and population sciences. Cancer survivorship research. Available at: http://dccps.cancer.gov/ocs/prevalence/prevalence.html. Accessed December 15, 2007. Data source: Ries LAG, Melbert D, Krapcho M, et al, editors. SEER cancer statistics review, 1975–2004. Bethesda (MD): National Cancer Institute, http://seer. cancer.gov/csr/1975_2004/, based on November 2006 SEER data submission, posted to the SEER web site, 2007.)

which represents a threefold increase from the 3 million prevalence estimate calculated for 1971 (see Fig. 1). Of these 10.8 million, 6.8 million (63%) had survived more than 5 years beyond their original diagnosis, 4.2 million (39%) were survivors of 10 or more years, and an impressive 1.5 million (14%) were diagnosed 20 or more years earlier (Fig. 2). In the absence of other competing causes, survival estimates for adults diagnosed with cancer indicate that 66% can expect to be alive in 5 years. These figures are even higher for those diagnosed as children (younger than 19 years of age) for whom 5-year survival is approaching 80% and 10-year survival is close to 75%. These numbers are in sharp contrast to the earlier period (1974–1976) when 5-year survival was only 50% for adults and 56% for children treated for cancer. Provided that current trends in incidence and mortality continue, it is expected that we will reach the cancer control goal established in the *Healthy People 2010* document of 70% 5-year survival for all those diagnosed with cancer in this country [15].

The lengthening prospect for survival is credited in large measure to advances in screening for many cancers, such as breast, cervical, and prostate cancer, and progress in the discovery, development, and delivery of more effective treatments for many cancers. These advances raise, nonetheless, a cautionary

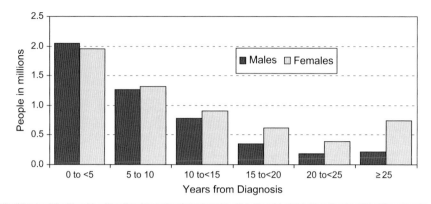

Fig. 2. Estimated number of people alive in the United States diagnosed with cancer on January 1, 2004 by time from diagnosis and gender (invasive/first primary cases only, N = 10.8 million). (*From* National Cancer Institute. Cancer control and population sciences. Cancer survivorship research. Available at: http://dccps.cancer.gov/ocs/prevalence/ prevalence.html. Accessed December 15, 2007. Data source: Ries LAG, Melbert D, Krapcho M, et al, editors. SEER cancer statistics review, 1975–2004. Bethesda (MD): National Cancer Institute, http://seer.cancer.gov/csr/1975_2004/, based on November 2006 SEER data submission, posted to the SEER web site, 2007.)

note. Specifically, current prevalence estimates, coupled with the emerging evidence regarding late and long-term medical and psychosocial health consequences of cancer and its treatment, highlight the importance of long-term follow-up and surveillance of the cancer survivor population [16–18]. With more individuals expected to live long term following their cancer treatment, the previously documented risk for subsequent cancers, including multiple primary breast cancers in female breast cancer survivors, the increased incidence of thyroid cancer after prostate cancer, or elevated risk for subsequent colon cancer in patients who have colorectal cancer, is beginning to raise concern for the long-term health of this population [19,20]. At present, roughly 16% of new cancer cases diagnosed annually occur in individuals who are already cancer survivors [20].

With respect to cancer history, breast cancer survivors have historically and continue to represent the largest segment of the survivor population (23%) followed by prostate cancer survivors (19%) and colorectal cancer survivors (10%) (Fig. 3). Among female survivors, cancers of the breast (42%), corpus and uterus (10%), and colon and rectum (9%) account for almost two thirds (61%) of prevalent cases. Cancers of the prostate (41%), colon and rectum (11%), and hematologic sites (9%) are the most prevalent cases in male survivors [14]. Consonant with their higher incident rates of cancer, there are more men than women within 5 years of diagnosis. More women than men become long-term (>5 years) survivors, however, because of higher proportions of women having more easily diagnosed and controlled cancers (eg, breast and gynecologic), lower incidence and mortality from lung cancer

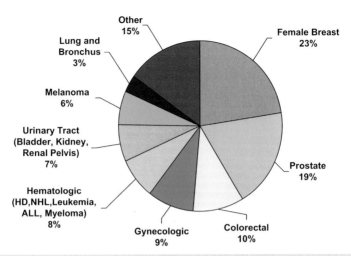

Fig. 3. Estimated number of people alive in the United States diagnosed with cancer by cancer site (invasive/first primary cases only, N = 10.8 million). (*From* National Cancer Institute. Cancer control and population sciences. Cancer survivorship research. Available at: http://dccps. cancer.gov/ocs/prevalence/prevalence.html. Accessed December 15, 2007. Data source: Ries LAG, Melbert D, Krapcho M, et al, editors. SEER cancer statistics review, 1975–2004. Bethesda (MD): National Cancer Institute, http://seer.cancer.gov/csr/1975_2004/, based on November 2006 SEER data submission, posted to the SEER web site, 2007.)

(although in contrast to men's, women's rate of lung cancer mortality continues to increase, reflecting historic gender differences in adoption of smoking behavior) [13], and generally lower all-cause mortality rates among women as compared with men in the United States. To the extent that women continue to pursue lifestyles and behaviors more similar to their male counterparts that put them at greater risk for cancer (eg, smoke, drink, sunbathe, live and work in toxic environments, and fail to exercise regularly), their gender advantage in long-term survivorship may well diminish over time.

Survivors who are 19 years of age or younger compose only 1% of the prevalent cancer population (10.8 million). Young adults who have cancer (20–39 years of age) represent 5% of the cancer survivor population, whereas survivors 40 to 59 years of age account for 24% of the population. Notably, men and women older than the age of 60 years who have a history of cancer represent the largest segment (70%) of the survivor population, reminding us of the intimate relationship between aging and cancer (Fig. 4). The median age at cancer diagnosis, based on Surveillance, Epidemiology, and End Results (SEER)–17 was 67 years; overall, 56% of new cases were diagnosed in patients 65 years and older [21]. For some cancers, these latter rates are even higher (eg, colorectal, 72%; lung, 68%; prostate, 64%). With fewer deaths from cardiovascular disease and broader diffusion into the community of advances in cancer detection, treatment, and care, the number of survivors will continue to

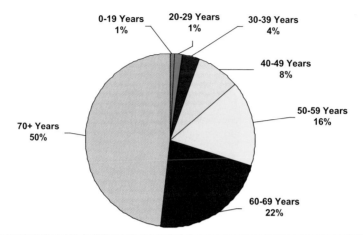

Fig. 4. Estimated number of people alive in the United States diagnosed with cancer by current age. (invasive/first primary cases only, N = 10.8 million). (*From* National Cancer Institute. Cancer control and population sciences. Cancer survivorship research. Available at: http://dccps.cancer.gov/ocs/prevalence/prevalence.html. Accessed December 15, 2007. Data source: Ries LAG, Melbert D, Krapcho M, et al, editors. SEER cancer statistics review, 1975–2004. Bethesda (MD): National Cancer Institute, http://seer.cancer.gov/csr/1975_2004/, based on November 2006 SEER data submission, posted to the SEER web site, 2007.)

increase. An even more powerful force in determining the face of tomorrow's survivors, however, is the aging of the nation's—indeed the world's—population.

A LOOK AT TOMORROW'S SURVIVORS

Age remains the single most important risk factor for cancer. The profile of cancer survivors is thus expected to change in parallel with the major shifts taking place in the age structure of the United States population attributable largely to the aging of the "baby boomer" cohort. Men and women older than 65 years of age represent 12% (36.8 million) of the United States population and this portion of the United States population is expected to double by the year 2030; 40% will be from minority groups [22]. The fastest-growing segment of the population is the oldest old, those aged 85 years and over. Projections suggest the oldest old will increase from 3.7 million in 1996 to 5.7 million in 2010 and could reach 18.2 million by 2050 [22,23]. Fig. 5 depicts the projected pattern of cancer incident counts between the years 2000 and 2050 by age group. These estimates suggest that the number of men and women aged 65 years and older diagnosed with cancer will double by 2050, assuming incident rates remain the same or do not increase [23]. As a result, the number of older cancer survivors will increase at an even greater rate putting unprecedented demands on the health care system.

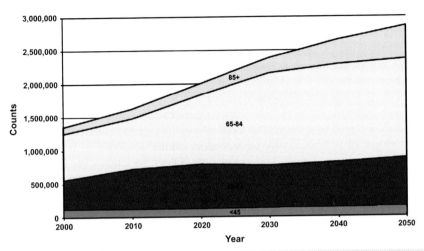

Fig. 5. Projected pattern of incident counts for 2000 to 2050 by age group (<45, 45–64, 65–84, 85+) based on projected census population estimates and delay-adjusted SEER-17 cancer incidence rates. Projections based on approximate single-year delay adjusted SEER-17 incidence rates for 1998 to 2002 and population projections from the U.S. Census Bureau. (*Data from* Edwards BK, Howe HL, Ries LA, et al. Annual report to the nation on the status of cancer, 1973–1999, featuring implications of age and aging on U.S. cancer burden. Cancer 2002;94(10):2766–92.)

Currently, 60% of all incident malignancies in the United States occur in adults older than the age of 65 years and 16% of those older than 65 years have a history of cancer [14]. Although cancer is the second leading cause of death among men and women aged 65 or older [22], numerous older adults are surviving cancer. In the United States alone, it is estimated that 6.5 of the 10.8 million cancer survivors are 65 years of age or older with the oldest old composing 15% of this 6.5 million. Forty-three percent of the 6.5 million older men and women were more than 10-year survivors of their disease; 17% had survived more than 20 years beyond their initial diagnosis [14]. These estimates suggest many older adults who have cancer live with, instead of die from, cancer and its treatments.

Not surprisingly, the cancer and aging interface has emerged as an important area of inquiry for oncology clinicians and geriatricians as reflected by a recent Institute of Medicine workshop on cancer in the elderly and a special issue of the *Journal of Clinical Oncology* on this topic [24,25]. Most of that attention is focused on treatment issues, particularly exploring the interplay of comorbidities, extent of treatment offered, efficacy of treatment, and prognostic outcomes. This is only part of the picture of the relationship of cancer and aging, however. The most neglected side of past attempts at understanding the cancer and aging interface is understanding the longer-term survivorship experience and needs of older cancer survivors [26,27].

Unfortunately, evidenced-based practice guidelines regarding posttreatment care for this group are sparse and it would be inappropriate to extrapolate recommendations for care from extant studies on younger populations, because older adults are physiologically, psychologically, and socially different than younger adults [27–30]. Unlike younger adults, the experience of cancer in the elderly is often superimposed on existing health conditions, including heart disease, arthritis, diabetes, and various geriatric syndromes that affect older adults [31–33]. These coexisting medical conditions can complicate the efficacy and extent of treatment offered and older adults' response to treatment and their downstream health and well-being. Older patients who have cancer tend to be in poorer health (34% versus 10% of the general population), are more likely to have two or more chronic medical conditions (16% versus 4%), report significantly more functional limitations (70% versus less than 30%), and experience greater limitations in activities of daily living (eg, bathing, dressing, eating) and instrumental activities of daily living (eg, cooking, cleaning house, shopping) (17% versus 3%) [34].

Given this emerging picture, it is clear that planning for the health care needs of our aging population, many of whom will be already, or become as they age, long-term cancer survivors, represents a significant public health challenge for the future. Our ability to successfully manage this new demand will rest in no small measure on our capacity to structure, conduct, and assess the impact of care informed by high-quality survivorship research.

SURVIVORSHIP RESEARCH: TRENDS AND LESSONS

Survivorship research is not new. Early efforts in this area are well chronicled by others [35–38]. Arguably, however, this field of study did not truly come of age until it was officially recognized as a part of the formal cancer control continuum, a topic warranting attention of its own. This turning point may be seen as having occurred when, in 1996, the Office of Cancer Survivorship (OCS) was established at the National Cancer Institute (NCI). The office was created in direct response to the articulate and compelling demand by the broader cancer advocacy community for a better understanding of the unique and poorly understood needs of those living with, through, and beyond cancer. Its establishment reflected the belief by NCI leadership that these concerns should be part of the institute's broader mandate or purview of research. The overall mission of the OCS is to enhance not only the length but also the quality of life of those diagnosed with cancer. In particular, the OCS was expected to champion research among those living long term (5 or more years) postdiagnosis. As defined by OCS, survivorship research seeks to: identify and control adverse cancer- and treatment-related outcomes (such as pain, lymphedema, sexual dysfunction, second cancers, and poor quality of life); provide a knowledge base regarding optimal follow-up care and surveillance of cancer survivors; and optimize health after cancer treatment (http://cancercontrol.cancer.gov/ocs/definitions.html). The function of survivorship research can be seen as five-fold. Information about survivors' anticipated health and well-being is critical if we are to: help patients make decisions now about treatment options that will affect their future; understand the action of, and as needed modify, therapies to maximize cure while minimizing adverse treatment-related effects; develop and disseminate evidence-based interventions that reduce cancer morbidity and mortality and facilitate adaptation among cancer survivors; improve quality of care and control costs; and equip the next generation of physicians, nurses, and other health care professionals to deliver not just the science but also the art of comprehensive cancer medicine [38].

In 1998, when it was moved into the newly established Division of Cancer Control and Population Sciences at NCI, the OCS had oversight of only 9 grants. Today, the scientific staff manages more than 150 grants, bearing witness to the lesson that "if you build it, they will come." Over time, the nature of the research being funded has evolved also. Early studies among survivors were often conducted in the setting of a single institution (frequently a major cancer center), by a limited number of investigators representing only a few disciplines; they tended to be atheoretical in design and were largely descriptive in nature. Over time survivorship studies have become more sophisticated in the science they propose, diverse with respect to the populations examined, and complex with regard to the multidisciplinary leadership; teams and often multiple study sites are involved, and in content they have come to span the cancer research continuum from basic or bench science (eg, examining the relationship between molecular markers of DNA repair and recurrence in Hodgkin lymphoma), to bedside (eg, telephone counseling for head and neck cancer survivors; acupuncture for hot flashes), to community (eg, Internet-delivered peer support for breast cancer; strength training for survivors delivered through Cooperative Community Oncology Program partners).

To track the success and direction of the work being pursued in cancer survivorship research, the OCS conducts annually (starting in 2001) an informal NIH-wide analysis of grants that address the posttreatment period of the cancer control continuum. In the most recent analysis, reviewing funding for fiscal year 2006, a total of 251 grants were identified. (http://cancercontrol.cancer.gov/ocs/analysis2006.html). Although most of these are housed within NCI (N = 220, 88%), several other institutes also fund research in this area, most notably the National Institute of Nursing Research, National Center for Complementary and Alternative Medicine, National Institute on Aging, National Institute for Mental Health, and the National Heart, Lung and Blood Institute.

Most grants continue to be descriptive or analytic studies (N = 129, 52%). Increasingly, however, the investigator community is moving into the arena of intervention research (N = 86, 34%). Long a paradigm for the study of the human impact of cancer survivorship [39], breast cancer and breast cancer survivors continue to be the sole focus of, or constitute a significant representation within, the sampling of most studies (N = 103). The next two populations of specific interest include survivors of hematologic malignancies (N = 43) or prostate cancer (N = 24), a distant second and third by comparison. As shown in Fig. 6, the characteristics of the populations being studied are

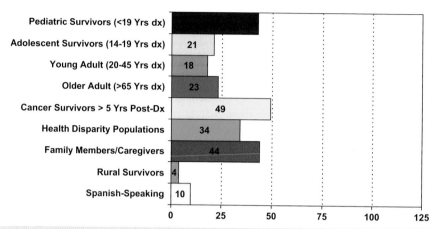

Fig. 6. Number of NIH survivorship research grants and cooperative agreements by study population (fiscal year 2006). Grants may have more than one focus.

becoming quite diverse; this is also true of the target long-term and late effects being monitored and addressed (Fig. 7).

The large number of grants that incorporate measures to assess or treat psychologic distress mirrors the historic emphasis on addressing individuals' and family members' adaptation to illness, recovery, and an uncertain future. At

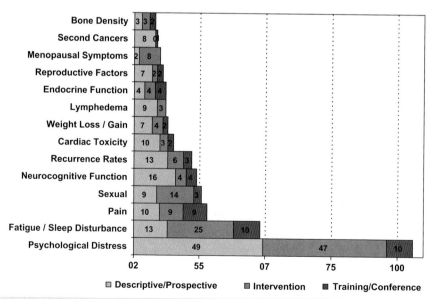

Fig. 7. Number of NIH survivorship grants and cooperative agreements by late/long-term effect (fiscal year 2006). Grants may have more than one focus.

one time this was the narrow extent of survivorship research. But also reflected in these data is the attention being paid to some of the more persistent effects of treatment (eg, fatigue, memory problems, weight gain), along with emerging problems associated in many cases with newer therapies, such as taxanes, aromatase inhibitors, or growth factors. Focus on specific topics is increasingly a function of survivors' accounts of problems in these domains (eg, lingering fatigue, sexual dysfunction), or clinicians' concerns about potential late sequelae (eg, cardiac failure, osteoporosis, second malignancies).

What is this science, or more accurately, what are survivors themselves telling us? First, as reflected in the other contributions to this special issue, being told they are disease free does not mean that survivors are truly free of their disease. Cancer has the capacity to affect all aspects of an individual's life: physical, psychologic, social, economic, and existential. Some of cancer's effects are acute and resolve quickly once treatment ends (eg, alopecia, nausea, anemia). Others, however, can be more insidious; they may persist over time and become long-term or chronic problems (eg, fatigue, cognitive problems, neuropathic pain syndromes, sexual dysfunction, body image changes). Still other, or late, effects may not show up until months or years after active treatment ends (eg, cardiovascular disease, osteoporosis, second malignancies). Survivors of all ages may be adversely affected, and although some experience few effects, others suffer multiple complications. As well chronicled in the two Institute of Medicine reports on survivorship [1,2], cancer's adverse sequelae contribute significantly to the personal and social burden of illness. At present, the degree of risk to any given patient of experiencing one or several of these is often difficult to predict. Although fear of recurrence and the risk for second cancers are often of most concern to survivors and their health care providers [40], other comorbid conditions, especially among older survivors, may be of greater concern as a threat to longevity [18,34,41].

Second, despite its potential for adverse consequences, the cancer experience is not all bad. Cancer survivors teach us time and again of the remarkable resilience of the human spirit [42]. While struggling with the negatives, survivors often report finding positive aspects of their ordeal [43–46]. There can be a profound sense of accomplishment on completion of an arduous course of therapy, of improved self-esteem at having mastered a difficult challenge. Grateful to be alive, many survivors express an enhanced appreciation for life, for each new day, and for those who helped them get through their treatments. This realization spawned in the past several years several studies examining cancer-related posttraumatic stress on the one hand [47–49] and posttraumatic growth or benefit finding on the other [44,45].

Third, cancer for many represents a "teachable" moment [50–52]. Research among survivors finds that many, struggling to take back control of their bodies and lives, are interested in and striving to make changes in their lifestyles and behaviors in the hopes that this might lessen the risk for new or recurrent disease [53,54]. Studies that examine or seek to intervene with respect to the health behaviors of survivors represent a fast-moving area within the current survivorship research portfolio. In fiscal year 2006, 31 studies fell into this category.

Fourth, cancer survivorship research, originally conceptualized as simply mapping the terrain of survival, has expanded rapidly beyond this more limited scope. It has even outgrown its small section on the linear cancer control continuum (eg, prevention, detection, treatment, survivorship, end of life). Clinicians and researchers have come to realize that research in this arena has the capacity to affect issues along the entire continuum. For example, the young adult breast cancer survivor, afforded the prospect of growing old with this history, must be counseled with regard to risk for (primary prevention) and screened for (secondary prevention) other cancers for which she would be at risk across the course of her life. Lengthening survivorship calls for a new model for thinking about research and care into the future (Fig. 8).

Fifth, and in many respects the most sobering lesson learned, no matter how quickly the research is moving or building, we are always a step behind the data. One of the key challenges to conducting cancer survivorship research is that the treatments are constantly changing. New drugs, new combinations of these, and new ways to deliver them will require continuous efforts to evaluate the potential for chronic or latent toxicities among newer generations of survivors. There will be new issues related to different psychosocial and economic problems generated by these changes. For example, with the shift to greater use of oral cancer medications, questions are arising about survivors' willingness to adhere to recommended regimens, especially if this involves long-term use and having to self-monitor and manage potential side effects. Although it is expected, or at least a hoped-for outcome, that the greater use of molecularly targeted agents combined with the push toward tailoring or personalizing therapy will result in fewer toxicities, history has taught us that there are no truly benign drugs; few if any agents are devoid of side effects. New

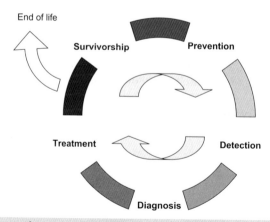

Fig. 8. Cancer control continuum (revisited).

tools and techniques to monitor and evaluate cancer's impact on individuals, their families, and society over time are clearly needed.

Taken as a whole, the growing body of high-quality survivorship research makes it clear that a focus on cure is no longer enough if we are to truly advance the science and art of cancer medicine. We have entered a new era in which the person must become as important, if not more important, than the tumor when planning, delivering, and monitoring the outcome of modern cancer care.

RESEARCH CHALLENGES FOR THE FUTURE

With more people living longer with a history of cancer, the need to identify those at increased risk for complications of treatment, and interventions to reduce that risk, is becoming increasingly urgent. Access to information about treatment-related risks is also critical if we are to help patients and their providers negotiate the treatment decision-making process. Central to any program of cancer survivorship research is always the need to identify and direct descriptive and analytic epidemiologic studies of cancer's long-term and late effects now and in the future. At the same time, a parallel body of research to develop, test, and deliver interventions designed to prevent or mitigate the adverse effects of having and being treated for cancer must also be supported.

A major hurdle to advancing work in these larger areas is the fast pace of change occurring in what types of and how cancer therapies are delivered. What may have been a significant concern for one cohort of survivors may be of little concern for the next generation treated. For example, understanding and helping colon cancer survivors deal with the physical, emotional, and social toll of undergoing a colostomy was a major focus of early survivorship research within this population. Today, with earlier diagnosis and new function-sparing surgical approaches to curing colon cancer, fewer patients face or undergo these procedures. The result is that attention to colostomy's impact has markedly diminished. Finding a balance between the need to identify emerging chronic and late effects of newer therapies and elucidating and treating the longer-term impact of older ones constitutes a fundamental challenge for the survivorship research community.

Beyond these major domains, there is a further set of specific areas in which we need to foster more research based on previously described gaps in current funding [38,55,56] and what has been identified as needed research in several of the national survivorship reports cited earlier [1–5]. These include:

(1) A focus on underserved and poorly studied populations of survivors. Several major national reports highlight the unequal burden of cancer faced by those from low-income backgrounds, diverse ethnocultural minorities, and rural communities [57–59]. New initiatives to address these health disparities must include research on the survivorship experience of many previously understudied groups. In addition, information about older survivors and those who have some of the most common malignancies (eg, colorectal cancer, gynecologic cancer, lymphoma) is also surprisingly limited [26,27]. Despite that more than half

(60%) of today's cancer survivors are aged 65 or older, and even higher proportions are expected to populate future survivor cohorts, only a fraction of our funded research is looking at the effect of cancer on these older Americans. Of the 251 grants funded in 2006, only 23 (less than 10%) specifically targeted survivors aged 65 or older. This segment of our nation's population is among the fastest growing. With the first of group of those born between the years of 1946 and 1964 turning 65 in 2011, we are going to see the baby boom generation enter the "cancer boom" era and need to move quickly to prepare to meet this impending challenge. Although there are some common normative processes that occur with advancing age, older adults are increasingly heterogeneous in their physical and psychosocial health as a result of previous lifestyle factors, environmental exposure, genetic makeup, and style of (and resources for) coping [60]. As a result, examining within-group and between-group differences is critical if we are to understand the posttreatment burden of this increasingly diverse population. Several areas of research warrant attention, including characterizing the posttreatment burden of disease in the older cancer survivor population, assessing the validity and reliability of commonly used health outcome instruments in the elderly, exploring the extent to which cancer may accelerate the aging process, and characterizing patients' changing illness and treatment representations (ie, expectations and beliefs) with age and its influence on care seeking, functioning, and quality of life.

(2) Attention to economic outcomes, patterns of care, and service delivery. Determining the cost, both personal and social, of cancer on individuals, their families, and society at large remains a challenge. Research is needed on the impact of cancer on work, economic status, and insurability, and on the impact that patterns of follow-up care have on survivors' health status, morbidity, and mortality. Devising strategies to compare the costs and benefits of different models of delivering posttreatment care to survivors will be a significant issue as we look to the future. Do cancer survivors have better health outcomes if they are seen in a specially staffed cancer survivors' clinic versus by their primary care physician? Could we reduce medical and human costs (associated with travel to and use of specialists) and still get good survivorship outcomes if we provide remote or on-line expert consultation to primary care physicians about best practices with respect to survivors' follow-up care? At the same time, we need to have a clearer understanding of the cost of delivery of many of the interventions that are found to improve quality of life and the functioning of survivors posttreatment. Because this type of health services research adds significantly to the expense of conducting a typical behavioral intervention study (eg, to reduce fatigue, promote coping, address sexual dysfunction), it is often omitted. As a consequence, the number of interventions in which this type of data is available are few and far between [61].

(3) A focus on family. Although caregivers are viewed by the advocacy community as encompassed under the definition of cancer survivors (http://dccps.nci.nih.gov/ocs), albeit secondary survivors, we are only just beginning to appreciate the impact cancer has on the functioning and well-being of the millions of family members affected by this illness, many of whom may themselves be at increased risk for cancer because of shared cancer-causing genes, lifestyle, or toxic exposures. With most cancer care delivered on an outpatient basis, and as survivors live longer, the burden on family of providing support for a loved one over the

course of his or her illness and recovery is growing. It is well known that social support is an important buffer to negative health outcomes [62–64]. Research is beginning to show that intervening with cancer caregivers may improve not only patients' but also caregivers' health outcomes [65–68].

(4) Instrument development. The past 2 decades saw the introduction of a host of well-developed tools to describe the impact of cancer diagnosis and treatment on individuals' health-related quality of life. As survivors live longer and age, however, new instruments are needed that enable us not only to more accurately describe the late effects of treatment but also to compare the well-being of those living with a history of cancer to that of their similarly aging peers who do not have such a history [69]. Tools that allow us to capture easily and early in the course of care (ideally before treatments start) information on conditions that may have predated illness onset and track this over time through periodic assessment also need to be developed. Several activities currently underway will help us achieve this goal. These include a growing emphasis on use of patient-reported outcomes in the setting of clinical trials [70]; development of efficient, valid, and reliable tools to collect this information [71]; efforts to reach consensus on comorbidity assessment [72,73]; and the movement, albeit frustratingly slow, toward universal adoption of electronic health records.

(5) Dissemination and diffusion. As we learn more about the cancer survivorship experience and the interventions or care needed to optimize outcomes, we must find ways to communicate this knowledge to those most in need of this information. The science of communication is growing quickly, in particular in the vital area of patient–doctor communication [74]. Whether we can become better at applying what we already know (something many lament we are failing to do) remains to be seen. At the same time, we need to mentor and train the next generation of clinicians and researchers to develop, study, and deliver state-of-the-art cancer care. This latter goal may prove to be more difficult to achieve than previously considered given the current climate of declining research budgets, shrinking tenure slots at major universities, as yet only modest investment in training programs in survivorship research and clinical practice, and anticipated shortages in not only oncology practitioners but also geriatricians and nurses [75,76]. It is clear that if we are to understand the complex interplay of genes-environment-behavior-society that affect survivors' outcomes, a premium will be placed on the ability to promote team science, or true transdisciplinary collaboration [77]. The continued emphasis on principal investigator status as a condition for academic advancement may thus prove a further hindrance to recruiting and retaining new cadres of clinical researchers.

As the field of cancer survivorship continues to mature, the final challenge we face is finding ways to measure the impact of our success. It is not enough to know that more people are surviving cancer or that more scientists and health care professionals are studying survivors' outcomes. We need to know that the research we are supporting is in fact improving the lives of these individuals and those who care for and about them. Among the questions we need to ask are: Can we use our surveillance systems to better describe the health status of the millions of survivors in this country now and tomorrow?

Our annually released prevalence figures tell us only how many individuals who have a cancer history are alive at a given point in time. They are silent with respect to the health status, quality of life, or place along the illness trajectory (eg, in treatment, posttreatment, living with, or dying from advanced disease) of the survivors counted. Plans for how to accomplish this have been delineated, but remain to be fully implemented [78]. How do we ensure that the interventions found successful in improving survivors' health outcomes can be and are adopted in the broader community? What should be the standards for care for cancer survivors who are posttreatment?

Benchmarks against which to measure progress already exist in other areas of cancer control. For example, change in smoking rates can be used to monitor the impact of primary prevention efforts, cancer screening uptake (eg, mammography, colonoscopy) among appropriate populations to determine the efficacy of secondary prevention campaigns, and survival curves to estimate more global success (or, as in the case of select minority populations, indicate places where improvement is needed) [13] in cancer control. A framework within which to assess improvements in quality cancer care has also been proposed [79]. By contrast, trends in survivorship outcomes, such as end-of-life care, remain relatively neglected. The question is, which benchmarks should be used to determine success in survivorship? [80] In monitoring survivors' experience should this information include prevalence of comorbid conditions in or level of health-related quality of life of survivor cohorts versus that for the general population, school achievement for childhood survivors, or job status or capacity for work in working-age adult survivors? Can and should we use survivors' health behaviors (eg, smoking, physical activity levels, cancer screening) to determine the impact of health promotion efforts, or medical care use as a means to evaluate the impact of supportive interventions? As these become formalized, assessing the uptake of follow-up care guidelines may serve as a quality indicator for monitoring our success in disseminating best practices for care (eg, development and delivery of treatment summaries and care plans; assessment of survivors for their psychosocial needs; delivery of care for noncancer conditions, such as diabetes and hypertension among survivors). Defining and achieving consensus around the specific metrics we will apply to measure our success in championing survivorship may well be the greatest and most important challenge for the decade to come.

In summary, as advances in cancer medicine turn this once uniformly fatal illness into a curable disease for growing numbers and a chronic illness for many, understanding and meeting the needs of long-term cancer survivors and their caregivers has become a major public health challenge, a challenge made more urgent by the aging of the population. The field of survivorship research, now moving into its adolescence, is helping document the long-term and late consequences of surviving cancer, and providing the evidence base for delivering interventions that will eliminate or reduce the adverse impact of illness and treatment on survivors and their families. As we look to the future, the need to fill the identified gaps in our knowledge base and keep up with changes in treatment and practice that lead to new gaps will continue to provide fundamental directions for research. We already have a great deal of information about what harms and helps people diagnosed with and treated for cancer, however. Providing care that conforms to this knowledge to survivors and their loved ones in all corners of the country must be an overarching goal. At the same time we need to find ways of identifying and applying methods to determine the impact we are having on reducing the burden of cancer for our growing population of survivors, their families, and society at large, to measure our success in achieving this ambitious, but critical, goal.

References

[1] Hewitt M, Weiner SL, Simone JV. Childhood cancer survivorship: improving care and quality of life. Washington, DC: The National Academies Press; 2003. Available at: http://www.nap.edu/catalog.php?record_id=10767.

[2] Hewitt M, Greenfield S, Stovall E. From cancer patient to cancer survivor: lost in transition. Washington, DC: Institute of Medicine and National Research Council of the National Academies; 2006. Available at: http://www.nap.edu/catalog.php?record_id=11468.

[3] Centers for Disease Control and Prevention (CDC), Lance Armstrong Foundation. A National action plan for cancer survivorship: advancing public health strategies. Atlanta (GA): U.S. Department of Health and Human Serivices, Center for Disease Control and Prevention; 2004. Available at: http://www.cdc.gov/cancer/survivorship/what_cdc_is_doing/action_plan.htm.

[4] President's Cancer Panel. 2003–2004 annual report. Living beyond cancer: finding a new balance. Bethesda (MD): National Cancer Institute; 2004. Available at: http://deainfo.nci.nih.gov/advisory/pcp/pcp03-04rpt/Survivorship.pdf.

[5] President's Cancer Panel. Assessing progress, advancing change. Bethesda (MD): National Cancer Institute; 2005.

[6] Rowland JH. Foreward: looking beyond cure: pediatric cancer as a model. J Pediatr Psychol 2005;30(1):1–3.

[7] Rowland JH, Hewitt M, Ganz PA. Cancer survivorship: a new challenge in delivering quality cancer care. J Clin Oncol 2006;24(32):5101–4.

[8] Aziz NM. Foreward: nursing and cancer survivorship. AJN 2006;106(3 Suppl):3.

[9] Feuerstein M. Handbook of cancer survivorship. New York: Springer; 2007.

[10] Ganz PA. Cancer survivorship: today and tomorrow. New York: Springer; 2007.

[11] Feuerstein M. Optimizing cancer survivorship. Journal of Cancer Survivorship 2007;1:1–4.

[12] Novack DH, Plumer R, Smith RL, et al. Changes in physician's attitudes toward telling the cancer patient. JAMA 1979;241:897–900.

[13] Espey DK, Wu XC, Swan J, et al. Annual report to the nation on the status of cancer, 1975–2004, featuring cancer in American Indians and Alaska natives. Cancer 2007;110(10):2119–52.

[14] Surveillance, Epidemiology, and End Results (SEER) Program (www.seer.cancer.gov). Prevalence database: "US Estimated Complete Prevalence Counts on 1/1/2004". National Cancer Institute, DCCPS, Surveillance Research Program, Statistical Research and Applications Branch, released April 2007, based on the November 2006 SEER data submission.

[15] U.S. Department of Health and Human Services. Healthy people 2010. With understanding and improving health and objectives for improving health. 2nd edition. Washington, DC: U.S. Government Printing Office; 2000.

[16] Aziz NM. Long-term survivorship: late effects. In: Berger AM, Portenoy RK, Weissman DE, editors. Principles and practice of palliative care and supportive oncology. Philadelphia: Lippincott Williams & Wilkins; 2002. p. 1019–33.

[17] Ganz PA, Desmond KA, Leedham B, et al. Quality of life in long-term, disease-free survivors of breast cancer: a follow-up study. J Natl Cancer Inst 2002;94(1):39–49.

[18] Oeffinger KC, Mertens AC, Sklar CA, et al. Chronic health conditions in survivors of childhood cancer. N Engl J Med 2006;355:1572–82.

[19] Hayat MJ, Howlader N, Reichman ME, et al. Cancer statistics, trends, and multiple primary cancer analyses from the Surveillance, Epidemiology, and End Results (SEER) Program. Oncologist 2007;12:1–20.

[20] Mariotto AB, Rowland JH, Ries LA, et al. Multiple cancer prevalence: a growing challenge in long-term survivorship. Cancer Epidemiol Biomarkers Prev 2007;16(3):566–71.

[21] Ries LA, Melbert D, Krapcho M, et al. SEER cancer statistics review, 1975–2004, National Cancer Institute. Available at: http://seer.cancer.gov/csr/1975_2004/ based on November 2006 SEER data submission, posted to the SEER web site; 2007.

[22] Centers for Disease Control and Prevention and The Merck Company Foundation. The state of aging and health in America 2007. Whitehouse Station (NJ): The Merck Company Foundation; 2007.

[23] Edwards BK, Howe HL, Ries LAG, et al. Annual report to the nation on the status of cancer, 1973-1999, featuring implications of age and aging on U.S. cancer burden. Cancer 2002;94(10):2766–92.

[24] Institute of Medicine. Cancer in elderly people. Workshop proceedings, National Cancer Policy Forum, Institute of Medicine. Washington, DC: The National Academies Press; 2007.

[25] Lichtman SM, Balducci L, Aapro M. Geriatric oncology: a field coming of age. J Clin Oncol 2007;25:1821–3.

[26] Rao AV, Demark-Wahnefried W. The older cancer survivor. Crit Rev Oncol Hematol 2006;60:131–43.

[27] Bellizzi KM, Rowland JH. The role of comorbidity, symptoms and age in the health of older survivors following treatment for cancer. Aging Health 2007;3:625–35.

[28] Boss GR, Seegmiller JE. Age-related physiological changes and their clinical significance. West J Med 1981;135(6):434–40.

[29] Baltes PB, Baltes MM. Psychological perspectives on successful aging: a model of selective optimization with compensation. In: Baltes PB, Baltes MM, editors. Successful aging: perspectives from the behavioral sciences. New York: Cambridge University Press; 1990. p. 1–34.

[30] Carstensen LL. Social and emotional patterns in adulthood: support for socioemotional selectivity theory. Psychol Aging 1992;7(3):331–8.

[31] Extermann M. Interaction between comorbidity and cancer. Cancer Control 2007;14(1):13–22.

[32] Balducci L. Aging, frailty, and chemotherapy. Cancer Control 2007;14(1):7–12.

[33] Hurria A. Clinical trials in older adults with cancer: past and future. Oncology 2007;21(3):351–8.

[34] Hewitt M, Rowland JH, Yancik R. Cancer survivors in the United States: age, health, and disability. J Gerontol A Biol Sci Med Sci 2003;58:82–91.

[35] Tross S, Holland JC. Psychological sequelae in cancer survivors. In: Holland JC, Rowland JH, editors. Handbook of psychooncology: psychological care of the patient with cancer. Oxford: Oxford University Press; 1989. p. 101–16.

[36] Kornblith AB. Psychosocial adaptation of cancer survivors. In: Holland JC, editor. Psycho-oncology. New York: Oxford University Press; 1998. p. 223–41.

[37] Meadows AT. Pediatric cancer survivors: past history and future challenges. Curr Probl Cancer 2003;27:112–26.

[38] Rowland JH. Survivorship research: past, present and future. In: Ganz PA, editor. Cancer survivorship today and tomorrow. New York: Springer; 2007. p. 28–42.

[39] Rowland JH. Psycho-oncology and breast cancer: a paradigm for research and intervention. Breast Cancer Res Treat 1994;31:315–24.

[40] Baker F, Denniston M, Smith T, et al. Adult cancer survivors: how are they faring? Cancer 2005;104(11):2565–76.

[41] Brown BW, Brauner C, Minnotte MC. Non cancer deaths in white adult cancer patients. J Natl Cancer Inst 1993;85:979–87.
[42] Aspinwall LG, MacNamara A. Taking positive changes seriously. Toward a positive psychology of cancer survivorship and resilience. Cancer 2005;104(11 Suppl):2549–56.
[43] Bellizzi KM, Miller MF, Arora NK, et al. Positive and negative life changes experienced by survivors of non-Hodgkin's lymphoma. Ann Behav Med 2007;34(2):188–99.
[44] Bellizzi KM, Blank TO. Predicting posttraumatic growth in breast cancer survivors. Health Psychol 2006;25(1):47–56.
[45] Stanton AL, Bower JE, Low CA. Posttraumatic growth after cancer. In: Calhoun LG, Tedeschi RG, editors. Handbook of posttraumatic growth: research and practice. Mahwah (NJ): Lawrence Erlbaum Associates; 2006. p. 138–75.
[46] Helgeson VS, Reynolds KA, Tomich PL. A meta-analytic review of benefit finding and growth. J Consult Clin Psychol 2006;74(5):797–816.
[47] Green B, Rowland J, Krupnick J, et al. Prevalence of posttraumatic stress disorder in women with breast cancer. Psychosomatics 1998;39:102–11.
[48] Vachon M. Psychosocial distress and coping after cancer treatment. Cancer Nurs 2006;29(2 suppl):26–31.
[49] Kangas M, Henry JL, Bryant RA. Posttraumatic stress disorder following cancer. A conceptual and empirical review. Clin Psychol Rev 2002;22(4):499–524.
[50] Demark-Wahnefried W, Aziz NM, Rowland JH, et al. Riding the crest of the teachable moment: promoting long-term health after the diagnosis of cancer. J Clin Oncol 2005;23(24):5814–30.
[51] Ganz PA. A teachable moment for oncologists: cancer survivors 10 million and growing. J Clin Oncol 2005;23:5458–60.
[52] Bellizzi KM, Rowland JH, Jeffery DD, et al. Health behaviors of cancer survivors: examining opportunities for cancer control intervention. J Clin Oncol 2005;23(34):8884–93.
[53] Demark-Wahnefried W, Pinto BM, Gritz ER. Promoting health and physical function among cancer survivors: potential for prevention and questions that remain. J Clin Oncol 2006;24(32):5125–31.
[54] Demark-Wahnefried W, Peterson B, McBride C, et al. Current health behaviors and readiness to pursue life-style changes among men and women diagnosed with early stage prostate and breast carcinomas. Cancer 2000;88:674–84.
[55] Aziz NM, Rowland JH. Trends and advances in cancer survivorship research: challenge and opportunity. Semin Radiat Oncol 2003;13:248–66.
[56] Cancer Survivorship. Moving beyond cure. Department of Health and Human Services. The National Institutes of Health. The National Cancer Institute report submitted in response to Senate Report 107–216, page 100, the Committee on Appropriations to Congress.
[57] Institute of Medicine. Crossing the quality chasm: A new health system for the 21st century. Washington, DC: National Academy Press; 2001.
[58] President's Cancer Panel Report. Voices of a broken system: real people, real problems. Bethesda (MD): National Cancer Institute; 2001.
[59] Institute of Medicine. The unequal burden of cancer. Washington, DC: National Academy Press; 1999.
[60] Whitbourne SK. The aging individual: physical and psychological perspectives. New York: Springer Publishing Company; 1996.
[61] Carlson LE, Bultz BD. Benefits of psychosocial oncology care: Improved quality of life and medical cost offset. Health Qual Life Outcomes 2003;17(1):1–8.
[62] Cohen S. Psychosocial models of the role of social support in the etiology of physical disease. Health Psychol 1988;7(3):269–97.
[63] Wortman CB. Social support and the cancer patient. Conceptual and methodologic issues. Cancer 1984;53(10 Suppl):2339–62.
[64] Kroenke CH, Kubzansky LD, Schernhammer ES, et al. Social networks, social support and survival after breast cancer diagnosis. J Clin Oncol 2006;24(7):1105–11.

[65] Northouse LL, Mood DW, Schafenacker A, et al. Randomized clinical trial of a family intervention for prostate cancer patients and their spouses. Cancer 2007;110(12): 2809–18.

[66] Northouse LL. Helping families of patients with cancer. Oncol Nurs Forum 2005;32(4): 743–50.

[67] Kurtz ME, Kurtz JC, Given CW, et al. Depression and physical health among family caregivers of geriatric patients with cancer: a longitudinal view. Med Sci Monit 2004;10(8):CR447–56.

[68] Kim Y, Baker F, Spillers RL, et al. Psychological adjustment of cancer caregivers with multiple roles. Psychooncology 2006;15(9):795–804.

[69] Fitzsimmons D. What are we trying to measure? Rethinking approaches to health outcome assessment for the older person with cancer. Eur J Cancer Care (Engl) 2004;13: 416–23.

[70] Clauser SB, Ganz PA, Lipscomb J, et al. Patient-reported outcomes assessment in cancer trials: evaluating and enhancing the payoff to decision making. J Clin Oncol 2007;25(32):5049–50.

[71] Ader D. Developing the Patient-Reported Outcomes Measurement Information System (PROMIS). Med Care 2007;45(5):S1–2.

[72] Yancik R, Ershler W, Satariano W, et al. Comorbidity: the ultimate geriatric syndrome. Report of the National Institute on Aging Task Force on Comorbidity. J Gerontol A Biol Sci Med Sci 2007;62(3):275–80.

[73] Lash TL, Mor V, Wieland D, et al. Methodology, design, and analytic techniques to address measurement of comorbid disease. J Gerontol A Biol Sci Med Sci 2007;62(3):281–5.

[74] Epstein RM, Street RLJ: Patient-centered communication in cancer care: promoting healing and reducing suffering. National Cancer Institute, NIH Publication No. 07-6225. Bethesda, MD; 2007.

[75] Erikson C, Salsberg E, Forte G, et al. Future supply and demand for oncologists: challenges to assuring access to oncology services. Journal of Oncology Practice 2007;3(2):79–86.

[76] Association of Directors of Geriatric Academic Programs. Geriatric medicine: a clinical imperative for an aging population, Part I. Annals of Long-Term Care 2005;13(3):18–22.

[77] Rosenfield PL. The potential of transdisciplinary research for sustaining and extending linkages between health and social sciences. Soc Sci Med 1992;35(11):1343–57.

[78] Wingo PA, Howe HL, Thun MJ, et al. A national framework for cancer surveillance in the United States. Cancer Causes Control 2005;16:151–70.

[79] Lipscomb J, Donaldson MS, Arora NK. Cancer outcomes research. J Natl Cancer Inst Monogr 2004;33:178–92.

[80] Ganz PA. What outcomes matter to patients: a physician researcher point of view. Med Care 2002;40(Suppl 6):III1–9.

Follow-up of Adult Cancer Survivors: New Paradigms for Survivorship Care Planning

Sandra J. Horning, MD

Stanford University, Stanford, CA, USA

The reality of cancer care in the twenty-first century is that patients live longer, the range of therapeutic options has markedly expanded, and patients are more likely to receive care from multiple providers, across diverse delivery systems, and over multiyear periods. In this context, it is a challenge for oncologists and hematologists and other health care providers to assemble the information needed to understand an individual's cancer treatment history to deliver optimal care. A common difficulty is extracting a coherent summary from a series of chronologically organized records from multiple sources. Without a summary available to them, patients who have experienced a series of complex treatments are not equipped to become partners in their own care.

It has been nearly 2 years since the Institute of Medicine (IOM) issued its report on adult cancer survivorship, *From Cancer Patient to Cancer Survivor: Lost in Transition* [1]. The report defined cancer survivorship as a distinct phase of cancer care (Fig. 1) for which awareness and improvement in quality was needed, particularly with regard to improved communication and planning. Prominent among the 10 recommendations of the IOM report was the routine provision of a treatment summary and a formal plan for survivorship care, to be explained to patients and shared among providers at the end of active cancer treatment. The President's Cancer Panel, the Centers for Disease Control and Prevention, and the Lance Armstrong Foundation have also strongly recommended and endorsed survivorship care planning [2,3].

Because formal written plans have not been integrated into the culture of cancer care, efforts to develop and assess such plans had to be developed. In recognition of the wide variability of challenges specific to individual survivors and the increasing complexity of multidisciplinary cancer care, personalization of survivorship plans is necessary. Despite the many practical barriers in providing an evidence-based, formalized plan, there has been progress toward achieving the goal of quality medical care for cancer survivors through the provision of templates for comprehensive care summaries and follow-up care plans as discussed here.

E-mail address: sandra.horning@stanford.edu

0889-8588/08/$ – see front matter
doi:10.1016/j.hoc.2008.01.005

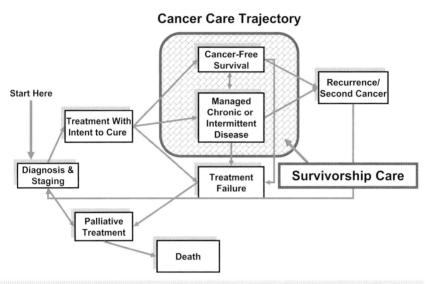

Fig. 1. The cancer care trajectory. (*From* Hewitt M, Greenfield S, Stovall E. From cancer patient to cancer survivors: lost in transition. Washington, DC: Institute of Medicine, National Academies Press; 2006; with permission.)

THE TREATMENT SUMMARY

Patients' understanding of their treatment plans and diagnoses vary widely at discharge from active treatment [4]. Cancer care, in particular, is complicated by the receipt of treatment from multiple providers, including medical and radiation oncologists, surgeons, other subspecialists, nurses, nutritionists, and psychosocial providers. Although organizations, such as the American Cancer Society and the Lance Armstrong Foundation, and institutions, such as the University of Washington and the University of Pennsylvania, have developed materials and Web sites to assist survivors in recording and summarizing their treatments, many patients are either not desirous or incapable of this task [5–7]. For this reason, it is essential that health care providers take on the responsibility for routinely providing a summary of treatment. Further, physicians who know the details of the treatment and its toxicity are in the best position to establish appropriate schedules for monitoring for recurrence and late effects and to guide referrals for ongoing problems.

Box 1 provides the basic elements of a summary at the end of active treatment. This record of care should, at a minimum, include: diagnostic tests performed and results; tumor characteristics, including stage and grade and biomarker information; details of surgery, chemotherapy, radiotherapy, hormonal therapy, and biotherapy; and identifying number and title of clinical trials. Indicators of treatment response and toxicities experienced should also be provided. The summary should include supportive services, such as psychosocial and nutritional services, and the full contact information for all key

Box 1: Components of a treatment summary: history of care

Diagnostic tests performed and results of tests

Tumor characteristics: site, stage, grade, biomarker information

Dates of treatment initiation and completion

Surgery, chemotherapy, radiotherapy, transplantation, hormonal therapy, bio-therapy, or other therapies provided, including agents used, treatment regi-men, total dosage, identifying number and title of clinical trials

Psychosocial, nutritional, and other supportive services provided

Full contact information of treating institutions and key individual providers

Identification of a key contact and a coordinator of continuing care

providers and treating institutions. Importantly, identification of a key point of contact and coordinator of continuing care should be stipulated.

More than simply a record of treatment, such a summary provides an opportunity for better communication with patients. In fact, preparation of a treatment plan document at the onset of treatment may lead to more optimal delivery of active cancer care. Such a synoptic document not only simplifies preparation of the later treatment summary but also enables the provider to organize and communicate the details of the cancer site, histology, and stage; goals of therapy and anticipated benefits; name and component drugs in the regimen; duration of treatment and number of planned cycles; strategy for assessing response; major side effects and precautions; and assessment of major risks, benefits, and reasonable alternatives. This document can be referred to throughout the period of active treatment.

As the American Society of Clinical Oncology (ASCO) moved forward with a group of dedicated oncologists from the community and academia to develop a template for a treatment summary, it became apparent that the variety of cancer types, therapeutic strategies, and goals made it difficult to develop a generic document. Rather, modifications must be tailored to circumstance. To date, ASCO has developed templates for adjuvant treatment of breast cancer (Fig. 2) and for colon cancer that are under evaluation in selected practices. These templates are available at http://www.asco.org and can be modified by practitioners. Ideally, the summary would be reviewed with the patient and family at the conclusion of treatment and made available to the primary care physician and other providers. As per the IOM recommendations, the treatment summary would go hand in glove with a survivorship care plan.

THE SURVIVORSHIP CARE PLAN

The IOM calls for a written plan for survivor care based on the best available evidence-based standards at the end of active treatment that is made available to patients and their primary health care providers. The elements of the care plan are given in Box 2.

Breast Cancer Adjuvant Treatment Plan and Summary v1.0 0907

[Insert Practice Name/Info Here]
The Treatment Plan and Summary is a brief record of major aspects of breast cancer adjuvant treatment. This is not a complete patient history or comprehensive record of intended therapies.

Medical oncology provider name:	
Patient name:	
Patient ID:	
Patient D.O.B:	(MM/DD/YY)
Age at diagnosis	
Patient phone:	
Support contact name:	
Support contact relationship:	
Support phone:	

Background Information			
Family history:	Click here to select		
Definitive breast surgery:	Date: (MM/DD/YY)	Type:	Click here to select
# of lymph nodes removed:	Click here to select		
# of lymph nodes positive:	Click here to select		
Axillary dissection: ☐ Yes ☐ No	If yes, enter date	(MM/DD/YY)	
Sentinel node biopsy: ☐ Yes ☐ No	If yes, enter date	(MM/DD/YY)	
Notable surgical findings/comments:			
Tumor type:	Click here to select		
Staging:	T stage - choose below	N stage - choose below	Pathologic stage - choose below
Oncotype DX recurrence score (if applicable):			
ER status:	Click here to select	PR status:	Click here to select
HER2 status:	Click here to select		
Major comorbid conditions:			
Echocardiogram or MUGA result prior to chemotherapy (if obtained):	EF= %		

Adjuvant Treatment Plan	**Adjuvant Treatment Summary**		
White sections to be completed prior to chemotherapy administration, shaded sections following chemotherapy			
Pre-treatment weight (lb/kg):	Post-treatment weight (lb/kg):		
Pre-treatment BSA:			
Date of last menstrual period: (MM/DD/YY)	Date of last menstrual period:	(MM/DD/YY)	
Name of regimen:			
Start date: (MM/DD/YY)	End date: (MM/DD/YY)		
Treatment on clinical trial: ☐ Yes ☐ No			
Chemotherapy Drug Name:	Dose reduction needed:	☐ Yes % ☐ No	
	Total # of cycles:		
Route			
Dose			
Schedule			
Chemotherapy Drug Name:	Dose reduction needed:	☐ Yes % ☐ No	
	Total # of cycles:		
Route			
Dose			
Schedule			
Chemotherapy Drug Name:	Dose reduction needed:	☐ Yes % ☐ No	
	Total # of cycles:		
Route			
Dose			
Schedule			
Chemotherapy Drug Name:	Dose reduction needed:	☐ Yes % ☐ No	
	Total # of cycles:		
Route			
Dose			
Schedule			

Fig. 2. Example of a treatment summary for early-stage breast cancer. (Reprinted with permission from the American Society for Clinical Oncology.)

Breast Cancer Adjuvant Treatment Plan and Summary v1.0 0907

Adjuvant Treatment Plan	Adjuvant Treatment Summary
Possible side effects of this regimen:	Anthracycline administered: ☐ Doxorubicin ____ mg/m2 ☐ Epirubicin ____ mg/m2
☐ Hair loss ☐ Fatigue	
☐ Nausea/Vomitting ☐ Menopause symptoms	Serious toxicities during treatment (list all below):
☐ Neuropathy ☐ Cardiac symptoms	
☐ Low blood count ☐ Other	
Reconstruction planned: ☐ Yes ☐ No	Hospitalization for toxicity during treatment: ☐ Yes ☐ No
If yes, date completed (MM/DD/YY)	
Radiation therapy planned: ☐ Yes ☐ No	Neurotoxicity that impairs activites of daily living: ☐ Yes ☐ No
If yes, date completed (MM/DD/YY)	
	Reason for stopping adjuvant treatment:

Endocrine Therapy	
Endocrine therapy planned: ☐ Yes ☐ No	Date endocrine therapy started (or to start):
Type - click here to select	(MM/DD/YY)
Medication:	
Duration:	

Trastuzumab (Herceptin) Therapy	
Trastuzumab (Herceptin) planned: ☐ Yes ☐ No	Trastuzumab (Herceptin) prescribed: ☐ Yes ☐ No
	Pre-trastuzumab ejection fraction: ___ % (MM/DD/YY)
	Most recent ejection fraction: ___ % (MM/DD/YY)
	Planned or completed dates of trastuzumab therapy Start date: (MM/DD/YY) End date: (MM/DD/YY)

Oncology Team Member Contacts	Survivorship Care Provider Contacts
Provider:	Provider:
Name:	Name:
Contact Info:	Contact Info:
Provider:	Provider:
Name:	Name:
Contact Info:	Contact Info:
Provider:	Provider:
Name:	Name:
Contact Info:	Contact Info:
Pre-treatment comments	Post-treatment comments

Fig. 2 (continued)

Box 2: Components of a written survivorship care plan

The likely course of recovery from treatment toxicities and the ongoing need for health maintenance of adjuvant treatment

A description of recommended cancer screening and other periodic testing and examinations, their schedule, and who should perform them

Information on possible late and long-term effects of treatment and symptoms of such effects

Information on possible signs of recurrence and second tumors

Information on the possible effects of cancer on marital/partner relationship, sexual functioning, work, and parenting, and the potential future need for psychosocial support

Information on the potential insurance, employment, and financial consequences of cancer and, as necessary, referral to counseling, legal aid, and financial assistance

Specific recommendations for healthy behaviors (eg, diet, exercise, healthy weight, sunscreen use, virus protection, smoking cessation, osteoporosis prevention)

As appropriate, information on genetic counseling and testing to identify high-risk individuals who could benefit from more comprehensive cancer surveillance, chemoprevention, or risk-reducing surgery

As appropriate, information on known effective chemoprevention strategies for secondary prevention

Referrals to specific follow-up care providers, support groups, or the patient's primary care provider

A listing of cancer-related resources and information (Internet-based sources and telephone listings for major cancer support organizations)

Fig. 3 provides an example of a survivorship care plan developed by ASCO volunteers and available on the Web sites http://www.asco.org and http://www.plwc.org. It is important to recognize the wide range of survivor needs at the conclusion of treatment and the requirement to individualize. For instance, some survivors have had definitive treatment with few side effects and wish to move on with their lives, whereas others have significant anxiety, distress, or ongoing health problems.

IMPLEMENTATION OF CANCER SURVIVORSHIP CARE PLANS

As a follow-up to the 2006 IOM report, the National Cancer Institute, National Coalition of Cancer Survivors, and the Lance Armstrong Foundation supported a workshop to implement survivorship care planning and conducted a focus group analysis of how a care plan could improve the quality of survivorship care [8,9]. This qualitative research revealed enthusiasm among survivors for such a plan and the receptiveness of primary care providers, who welcomed the plan and indicated their important role in the posttreatment period. Nurses emphasized the need to improve survivor care and that they could play an active

Breast Cancer Survivorship Care Plan v 1.0 09/07

Patient Name: ▓▓▓		Medical Oncologist Name: ▓▓▓	
FOLLOW-UP CARE TEST	**RECOMMENDATION**		**PROVIDER TO CONTACT**
Medical history and physical (H&P) examination (see below)	Visit your doctor every three to six months for the first three years after the first treatment, every six to 12 months for years four and five, and every year thereafter.		▓▓▓
Post-treatment mammography (see below)	Schedule a mammogram one year after your first mammogram that led to diagnosis, but no earlier than six months after radiation therapy. Obtain a mammogram every six to 12 months thereafter.		▓▓▓
Breast self-examination	Perform a breast self-examination every month. This procedure is not a substitute for a mammogram.		▓▓▓
Pelvic examination	Continue to visit a gynecologist regularly. If you use tamoxifen, you have a greater risk for developing endometrial cancer (cancer of the lining of the uterus). Women taking tamoxifen should report any vaginal bleeding to their doctor.		▓▓▓
Coordination of care	About a year after diagnosis, you may continue to visit your oncologist or transfer your care to a primary care doctor. Women receiving hormone therapy should talk with their oncologist about how often to schedule follow-up visits for re-evaluation of their treatment.		▓▓▓
Genetic counseling referral	Tell your doctor if there is a history of cancer in your family. The following risk factors may indicate that breast cancer could run in the family: • Ashkenazi Jewish heritage • Personal or family history of ovarian cancer • Any first-degree relative (mother, sister, daughter) diagnosed with breast cancer before age 50 • Two or more first-degree or second-degree relatives (grandparent, aunt, uncle) diagnosed with breast cancer • Personal or family history of breast cancer in both breasts • History of breast cancer in a male relative		▓▓▓

YEARLY BREAST CANCER FOLLOW-UP & MANAGEMENT SCHEDULE

| Visit Frequency for H&P Years 1-3: | ☐ 3 months | ☐ 6 months | *(check one)* |
| Years 4-5: | ☐ 6 months | ☐ 12 months | *(check one)* |

| Visit Frequency for Mammography: | ☐ 6 months | ☐ 12 months | *(check one)* |

VISIT FREQUENCY	**HISTORY AND PHYSICAL**	**MAMMOGRAPHY**
3rd **Month** (if applicable)	▓▓▓	
6th **Month** (if applicable)	▓▓▓	▓▓▓
9th **Month** (if applicable)	▓▓▓	
12th **Month** (if applicable)	▓▓▓	▓▓▓

Notes: ▓▓▓

• **Risk:** You should continue to follow-up with your physician because the risk of breast cancer returning continues for more then 15 years after remission.

• **Symptoms of Recurrence:** Report these symptoms to your doctor: new lumps, bone pain, chest pain, shortness of breath or difficulty breathing, abdominal pain, or persistent headaches.

• **Not Recommended:** The following tests are not recommended for routine breast cancer follow-up: breast MRI, FDG-PET scans, complete blood cell counts, automated chemistry studies, chest x-rays, bone scans, liver ultrasound, and tumor markers (CA 15-3, CA 27.29, CEA). Talk with your doctor about reliable testing options.

Fig. 3. Example of a survivorship care plan for early-stage breast cancer. (Reprinted with permission from the American Society for Clinical Oncology.)

role in creating and implementing survivorship care plans. Oncologists, although articulating support for the concept, were not inclined to complete survivorship care plans because of the burden of other reporting and communication requirements and limited time. Oncologists' attitudes and support, of course, must be addressed for care plans to become reality. It is hoped that a combination of patient demand, encouragement from medical schools and professional societies, reduction in burden through electronic health records, and reimbursement from insurance for their preparation and discussion will enable widespread adoption of survivorship care plans. It is also important to continue to further refine the templates and to formally evaluate their impact.

Although oncologists enjoy interacting and reassuring their cured patients, they must recognize that in many, if not most, cases patients may eventually elect or be forced to follow up with other care providers. The care plan provides their cherished patients with a permanent, "moveable" record that can accompany them whenever and wherever and should be made routine as a key element in quality cancer care. Further, the provision of a treatment summary is likely to have downstream benefits for oncologists and hematologists and their support staffs who become the recipients of care plans when called on to assume the care of patients who move or change insurers.

The care plans can only be as good as their contents and it is widely recognized that guidelines for surveillance for recurrence and complications of treatment are often lacking [1]. ASCO has published guidelines for two common conditions: surveillance of colorectal and breast cancer [10,11]. Intensive surveillance does not necessarily improve outcomes and, particularly with imaging, can lead to false-positive results, distress, and needless expense with subsequent investigations, and can even increase the risk for complications [12]. Although high-level evidence is rarely available, consensus recommendations can reduce variation in care. Consensus guidelines are provided for more than 100 tumor types by the National Comprehensive Cancer Network; these are estimated to cover ~95% of clinical circumstances [13]. The Children's Oncology Group developed comprehensive guidelines based on evidence if it exists and consensus if it does not [14]. Many of these recommendations are applicable to adults, particularly those treated as young adults.

An expert panel assembled by ASCO is working through a series of guidelines related to cancer survivorship. Guidelines for fertility preservation, an important consideration that must precede therapy for younger patients, have been published [15]. Although sufficient data were not available for guidelines for cardiac and pulmonary function monitoring, a systematic clinical review of the data was conducted and recently published [16]. Because of the difficulties in conducting survivorship research, incorporating follow-up for late effects or interventions to ameliorate late effects within the context of therapeutic clinical trials should be encouraged.

TEACHABLE MOMENTS

Consultation at the end of treatment has been described as a teachable moment to address healthy lifestyle and behaviors [17]. Specific recommendations for diet, exercise, smoking, immunizations, and genetic testing can be made. It is also an opportunity to recognize that comorbid conditions, particularly in older patients, must receive appropriate attention, as should screening recommendations for adults. Some data suggest that patients who have cancer, in fact, do not receive quality care for other chronic conditions [18]. The survivorship care plan can enlarge the scope of medical care beyond a narrow focus on the prior malignancy. The survivor care plan should be a dynamic document, frequently referred to in follow-up, providing multiple teachable moments and a compass for ongoing care and emphasis on wellness.

ADULT SURVIVORSHIP CARE

Survivorship care may represent the sequelae of curative cancer treatment or periods of managed intermittent or chronic cancer care (see Fig. 1). Although the value of a synopsis of treatment and care plan is obvious for patients who are transitioning back to non-oncology providers, treatment summaries and care plans are also likely to be useful for patients who have chronic malignancy undergoing complex multimodality therapy over extended periods. As indicated in Fig. 4, adapted from the IOM report, the largest number of ambulatory cancer care visits is with primary care providers. The new paradigm for cancer care survivor care must include shared educational opportunities and training, guidelines, and formalized care plans, with the inclusion of primary care physicians as part of a multidisciplinary team. To date, relatively little attention has been paid to the social and emotional challenges faced by survivors, who have real economic pressures in addition to their health problems. Survivors report general satisfaction with the clinical aspects of their care but frequently express dissatisfaction with oncologists' lack of attention to their psychologic needs [8]. Moving forward, survivorship care plans can provide an opportunity for discussion of nonmedical needs and referrals for ancillary services and expertise. In many cases, these needs represent areas beyond

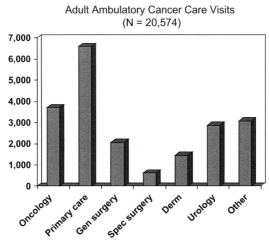

Adapted from Table 4-2, IOM Report, based on NAMCS, 2001-2002

Fig. 4. Ambulatory cancer care visits. (*From* Hewitt M, Greenfield S, Stovall E. From cancer patient to cancer survivors: lost in transition. Washington, DC: Institute of Medicine, National Academies Press; 2006; with permission.)

oncologists' capabilities but a list of resources available to patients and other providers, together with compassion and concern, can be invaluable.

Survivorship care plans should be dynamic documents that change with circumstances for individual patients and with the growth of knowledge and guidelines in specific relevant areas. The most important aspects of such plans are to openly communicate across the spectrum of survivor needs and concerns and to provide clarity for patients and providers. In the new paradigm, transitioning successful cancer care to healthy survivors becomes an integral part of every oncologist's education and practice.

References

[1] Hewitt M, Greenfield S, Stovall E. From cancer patient to cancer survivors: lost in transition Institute of Medicine. Washington, DC: National Academies Press; 2006.

[2] President's Cancer Panel. Living beyond cancer: finding a new balance. Bethesda (MD): National Cancer Institute; 2004.

[3] Centers for Disease Control and Prevention and Lance Armstrong Foundation. A national action plan for cancer survivorship: advancing public health strategies. Atlanta (GA): Centers for Disease Control and Prevention; 2004.

[4] Makaryus AN, Friedman EA. Patients' understanding of their treatment plans and diagnosis at discharge. Mayo Clin Proc 2005;80(8):991–4.

[5] Fred Hutchinson Cancer Research Center. Survivorship care plan. Available at: www.fhcrc. org/patient/support/survivorship/services/survive_care_plan.html. Accessed March, 2008.

[6] OncoLife survivorship care plan: Abramson Cancer Center of the University of Pennsylvania. Available at: http://www.oncolink.org/oncolife. Accessed March, 2008.

[7] Livestrong - Lance Armstrong Foundation: Cancer survivor's treatment summary. Available at: http://www.livestrong.org. Accessed March, 2008.

[8] Hewitt ME, Bamundo A, Day R, et al. Perspectives on post-treatment cancer care: qualitative research with survivors, nurses, and physicians. J Clin Oncol 2007;25(16):2270–3.

[9] IOM. Implementing cancer survivorship care planning: workshop summary. Washington, DC: National Academies Press; 2007.

[10] Khatcheressian JL, Wolff AC, Smith TJ, et al. American Society of Clinical Oncology 2006 update of the breast cancer follow-up and management guidelines in the adjuvant setting. J Clin Oncol 2006;24(31):5091–7.

[11] Desch CE, Benson AB III, Smith TJ, et al. Recommended colorectal cancer surveillance guidelines by the American Society of Clinical Oncology. J Clin Oncol 1999;17(4):1312–21.

[12] Brenner DJ, Hall EJ. Computed tomography—an increasing source of radiation exposure. N Engl J Med 2007;357(22):2277–84.

[13] National Comprehensive Cancer Network: Welcome to the NCCN Clinical Practice Guidelines in Oncology. Available at: http://www.nccn.org. Accessed March, 2008.

[14] Children's Oncology Group, Cure Search. Long-term follow-up guidelines for survivors of childhood, adolescent and young adult cancers. Available at: www.survivor shipguidelines.org. Accessed March, 2008.

[15] Nakayama K, Ueno NT. American Society of Clinical Oncology recommendations on fertility preservation should be implemented regardless of disease status or previous treatments. J Clin Oncol 2006;24(33):5334–5.

[16] Carver JR, Shapiro CL, Ng A, et al. American Society of Clinical Oncology clinical evidence review on the ongoing care of adult cancer survivors: cardiac and pulmonary late effects. J Clin Oncol 2007;25(25):3991–4008.

[17] Ganz PA. A teachable moment for oncologists: cancer survivors, 10 million strong and growing!. J Clin Oncol 2005;23(24):5458–60.

[18] Earle CC, Neville BA. Under use of necessary care among cancer survivors. Cancer 2004;101(8):1712–9.

Survivors of Childhood Cancer: Coming of Age

Melissa M. Hudson, MD[a,b,*]

[a]Department of Pediatrics, LeBonheur Children's Medical Center, University of Tennessee
College of Medicine, 50 North Dunlap, Room 306-307, TN 38103, USA
[b]Division of Cancer Survivorship, Department of Oncology, St. Jude Children's
Research Hospital, 332 North Lauderdale Street, Memphis, TN 38105, USA

Progress in cancer biology and therapeutics, radiologic sciences, and supportive care has produced increasing numbers of childhood cancer survivors who are living into adulthood. Presently, over 80% of children and adolescents with cancer survive 5 or more years from diagnosis and are effectively cured of the disease [1]. In the United States, this success represents almost 300,000 survivors, or 1 in 640 young adults between the ages of 20 and 39 years [2,3]. Unfortunately, the childhood cancer experience predisposes long-term survivors to a variety of chronic health problems [4,5], diminished health status including functional impairment and activity limitations [6–9], quality of life deficits and psychosocial disorders [10–14], and excess risk of early mortality [15]. Although advances in supportive care and therapeutic modifications undertaken over the last 30 years have significantly reduced the incidence of acute life-threatening events in children undergoing therapy for cancer, the impact of the cancer experience after contemporary therapy cannot be truly appreciated until achievement of long-term survival into adulthood. Lifelong follow-up of childhood cancer survivors is recommended to define accurately cancer-related morbidity, facilitate timely diagnosis of secondary disease, and implement remedial or preventive interventions that optimize health outcomes [16]. This article (1) provides readers with an appreciation of the scope of impact of childhood cancer on long-term survivor health, (2) underscores the need for ongoing risk-based monitoring after the cancer experience to optimize health outcomes and quality of life, (3) addresses the challenges in coordinating long-term survivor care, and (4) provides information

Dr. Hudson is supported in part by the Cancer Center Support (CORE) grant CA 21765 from the National Cancer Institute and by the American Lebanese Syrian Associated Charities (ALSAC).

*Division of Cancer Survivorship, Department of Oncology, St. Jude Children's Research Hospital, 332 North Lauderdale Street, Memphis, TN 38105. E-mail address: melissa.hudson@stjude.org

0889-8588/08/$ – see front matter
doi:10.1016/j.hoc.2008.01.011

about currently available health screening guideline resources that can be used to facilitate survivor care.

LATE EFFECTS: THE COST OF CURE

The cost of cure includes a spectrum of adverse effects that range from life-threatening to life-altering conditions. Although some complications are identified early in the clinical course following diagnosis and initiation of therapy, most do not manifest until years after completion of therapy. For example, in children, some cancer-related problems do not become apparent until growth and pubertal development are completed. Adults surviving childhood cancer may present with health issues resulting from their cancer therapy that have been exacerbated by organ dysfunction associated with aging and maladaptive health behaviors. Cancer-related complications that persist or develop 5 or more years after completion of cancer therapy, termed "late effects," are commonly reported in adults who have survived childhood cancer and demonstrate an increasing prevalence associated with longer time elapsed from cancer diagnosis [5]. Among 10,397 adult participants (mean age, 26.6 years) of the Childhood Cancer Survivor Study (CCSS), 73.4% will develop at least one chronic health problem by 40 years of age and over 40% will experience a chronic condition that is severe, life-threatening, or fatal [5]. Dutch investigators observed comparable rates of morbidity to that reported by the CCSS following comprehensive clinical evaluations of 1362 5-year survivors of childhood cancer (median age, 24.4 years): nearly 75% of survivors experienced one or more adverse events with 40% of events categorized as severe, life-threatening, or disabling [4]. Both studies linked specific treatment and host factors with the risk of particular adverse events, emphasizing the need for risk-stratified medical surveillance of childhood cancer survivors.

THE SPECTRUM OF LATE EFFECTS ASSOCIATED WITH CHILDHOOD CANCER

Growth and Development

The common late effects of pediatric cancer encompass several broad domains including growth and development, organ function, reproductive capacity and health of offspring, and development of subsequent neoplasms. Childhood cancer and its therapy may impact growth and development through adverse effects on linear growth, sexual maturation, musculoskeletal development, skeletal maturation, intellectual function, and emotional and social maturation [17,18]. Table 1 provides a summary of the specific late effects pertinent to this domain and predisposing childhood cancer therapies. Host factors, such as age and gender, modify the risk of these complications. In addition, specific diagnostic types are at higher risk because of the requirement for therapy that impacts the central nervous system (CNS). In general, younger age at treatment is associated with a higher risk of radiation-related injury to musculoskeletal tissues and adverse effects on linear growth [19–21]. The exception is that older age at diagnosis is associated with an increased risk of osteonecrosis predisposed by glucocorticoid

Table 1
Spectrum of effects on growth and development associated with pediatric cancer therapy

General domain	Specific late effect	Predisposing therapy	Modifying host factors
Linear growth	Delayed or accelerated growth	Radiation impacting hypothalamic-pituitary-growth hormone axis	Younger age at irradiation at higher risk
	Growth failure		
	Short stature		
Sexual maturation	Delayed or arrested puberty	Alkylating agents	Boys at higher risk of alkylating agent gonadal injury
	Early or precocious puberty	Radiation impacting hypothalamic-pituitary-gonadal axis	Girls at higher risk of early or precocious puberty
	Hypogonadism		
Musculoskeletal development	Hypoplasia	Radiation impacting bones and soft tissues	Younger age at irradiation at higher risk
	Fibrosis		
	Reduced or uneven growth (scoliosis, kyphosis, limb length discrepancy, and so forth)		
Skeletal maturation	Osteopenia	Corticosteroids	Both sexes at risk of bone mineral deficits
	Osteoporosis	Methotrexate	Younger age at irradiation at higher risk
		Radiation ($\geq$40 Gy) to skeletal structures	
	Osteonecrosis	Corticosteroids	Older age ($\geq$10 y) at treatment
Intellectual function	Neurocognitive deficits (executive function, memory, attention, processing speed, and so forth)	Methotrexate (high-dose intravenous or intrathecal)	Younger age at irradiation at higher risk
	Learning deficits	Cytarabine (high-dose intravenous or intrathecal)	
	Diminished IQ	Radiation impacting the brain	
	Behavioral problems		
Emotional and social maturation	Mental health disorders (depression, anxiety, posttraumatic stress, and so forth)	Any cancer experience	Girls and central nervous system tumor survivors at higher risk
	Educational problems		
	Vocational limitations		
	Underemployment or unemployment		
	Psychosocial disorders (difficulty with peer relationships, social withdrawal or isolation)		
	Limitations in health care and insurance access		

use [22]. Both sexes are at risk of bone mineral deficits associated with cancer treatment [23]. Girls are more predisposed to cognitive deficits after CNS-directed therapy, whereas boys are more sensitive to the effects of alkylating agents on gonadal function [24]. Because of local tumor effects, children with primary CNS tumors are particularly vulnerable to the adverse effects of cancer therapy on intellectual function and emotional-social maturation [25].

Organ Function

Table 2 summarizes the impact of pediatric cancer therapy on organ system function. Recognition of life-threatening effects on vital organ function (eg, anthracycline-induced cardiomyopathy) prompted modification of treatment protocols that eliminated or restricted exposure in patients with favorable disease presentations. Consequently, acute life-threatening vital organ toxicity involving the heart, lungs, liver, or kidneys rarely occurs following contemporary therapy. Subclinical cardiac injury has been reported, however, in a substantial proportion of survivors treated with anthracycline chemotherapy that may predispose to clinically symptomatic cardiac disease with increasing passage of time from therapy [26,27]. In contrast, the long-term implications of subclinical pulmonary dysfunction observed in association with contemporary cancer therapy have not been established. Current studies support that clinically significant pulmonary morbidity is limited to high-risk groups, such as survivors of hematopoietic cell transplant [28]. Urinary tract injury from such agents as cisplatin and ifosfamide has been significantly reduced by limiting cumulative dosage and routinely using uroprotectant agents and postchemotherapy hydration [29,30]. In contrast, toxic effects involving endocrine and neurosensory organs are still commonly observed, although the prevalence has been reduced with restriction of radiation doses and treatment fields and specific chemotherapeutic agents, such as cisplatin [21,31,32]. In general, exposure to higher cumulative chemotherapy and radiation doses as required for more biologically aggressive or refractory disease increases the risk of both vital and nonvital organ toxicity.

Reproductive Capacity and Pregnancy Outcomes

Reproductive health may be negatively impacted by a variety of anticancer modalities (Table 3). Surgical removal of the gonads (orchiectomy or oophoropexy) may affect fertility potential secondary to reduction in numbers or loss of germ cells. Pelvic surgery increases the risk of sexual dysfunction in both men and women treated for childhood cancer; these symptoms may be exacerbated in survivors with androgen or estrogen insufficiency [33,34]. Alkylating agent chemotherapy produces a dose-related risk of gonadal germ cell injury. In boys, alkylator-induced damage to germ cells resulting in infertility is very common, whereas Leydig cell function is typically preserved [35,36]. Compared with boys, girls maintain ovarian function at higher cumulative alkylating agent doses. The ovaries of prepubertal and adolescent girls are more resistant to alkylator-induced damage compared with adults because of their greater complement of follicles [35,36]. Most female childhood cancer patients treated with standard combination chemotherapy retain or recover ovarian function after completion of therapy. Treatment with higher cumulative doses (eg, dose-intensive alkylating agents for myeloablative conditioning before hematopoietic cell transplantation) is associated with a substantial risk of acute ovarian failure and premature menopause [37,38]. Combined modality therapy including alkylating agents and abdominal or pelvic radiation may also adversely impact fertility potential; CCSS investigators estimated a 30% cumulative incidence of nonsurgical menopause by age 40 in women who received this therapy [38].

Sperm production is reduced in a dose-dependent fashion following radiation. Azoospermia may be reversible at doses of 1 to 3 Gy, but is usually irreversible when doses exceed 3 Gy [35,36]. Prepubertal status does not protect from germ cell injury. Abdominal, pelvic, or spinal radiation may also contribute to germ cell depletion in girls [39,40]. Again, the ovaries of younger patients are more resistant to radiation injury than are those of older women. Radiation doses in excess of 20 Gy produce permanent ovarian failure in most female childhood cancer patients. Doses in the range of 20 to 30 Gy may delay or stall pubertal development.

For most childhood cancer survivors who maintain fertility, studies of health outcomes of offspring do not support an excess risk of birth defects or adverse pregnancy events [41,42]. The exception occurs in women treated with radiation impacting the uterus, which includes treatment fields to the whole abdomen, pelvic, lumbar or sacral spine, and total body [43]. Radiation-induced uterine vascular insufficiency has been linked to excess risk of spontaneous abortion, neonatal death, low-birth-weight infant, fetal malposition, and premature labor [40]. It should be noted that some of these complications are associated with congenital anomalies of the uterus that have been noted to be prevalent in 10% of girls with Wilms' tumor.

Subsequent Malignant Neoplasms

Childhood cancer survivors have an increased risk of developing second and subsequent cancers that varies by host factors (genetics, immune function, hormonal status); primary cancer therapy; environmental exposures; and lifestyle factors. Secondary carcinogenesis is likely multifactorial in etiology and results from combinations of influences including gene-environment and gene-gene interactions [44]. The histologic subtypes of second cancers encompass a neoplastic spectrum ranging from benign and low-grade malignant lesions to high-grade malignancies [45–51]. Outcome following diagnosis is variable; treatment for some histologic subtypes may be compromised if childhood cancer therapy included cumulative doses of agents and modalities at the threshold of tissue tolerance. Two broad histologic categories dominate (acute myeloid leukemia, including myelodysplastic syndrome, and solid tumors) as illustrated in Table 4, which summarizes standardized incidence ratios of second and subsequent malignancies reported by CCSS participants.

Secondary acute myeloid leukemia most commonly develops in association with alkylating agent or topoisomerase II inhibitor therapy [52,53]. The latency to onset is relatively brief: peak 5 to 10 years after alkylating agent therapy and

Table 2
Organ system dysfunction associated with pediatric cancer therapy

Organ system	Specific late effect	Predisposing therapy	Modifying host factors
Auditory	Sensorineural hearing loss Tinnitus Vertigo	Cisplatin Carboplatin Radiation impacting the ear	Younger age (<4 y) at treatment at higher risk
	Tympanosclerosis Otosclerosis Eustachian tube dysfunction Conductive hearing loss	Radiation impacting the ear	Younger age at treatment at higher risk
Cardiac	Cardiomyopathy Arrhythmias Subclinical left ventricular dysfunction	Anthracyclines (daunorubicin, doxorubicin, idarubicin, epirubicin)	Younger age (<5 y) at treatment at higher risk Girls at higher risk of anthracycline injury
	Congestive heart failure Cardiomyopathy Pericarditis Pericardial fibrosis Valvular disease Myocardial infarction Arrhythmia Atherosclerotic heart disease	Radiation impacting the heart	Younger age at irradiation at higher risk
Vascular	Carotid or subclavian artery disease Stroke Moyamoya Occlusive cerebral vasculopathy	Radiation impacting cardiovascular or cerebrovascular structures	History of Down syndrome, sickle cell disease, or neurofibromatosis
Endocrine and metabolic	Overweight or obesity Metabolic syndrome	Radiation impacting the brain	Younger age (<4 y) at treatment Girls at higher risk
	Hypothyroidism	Radiation impacting hypothalamic- pituitary axis Radiation impacting thyroid gland	Younger age at irradiation at higher risk Girls at higher risk

Organ system	Condition	Therapeutic exposures	Predisposing host factors
Hepatic	Chronic hepatitis C	Blood product transfusion before implementation of donor screening in 1992	History of chronic hepatitis B, HIV, or hematopoietic cell transplant
	Hepatic dysfunction	Methotrexate, Mercaptopurine, Thioguanine	History of chronic hepatitis
	Veno-occlusive disease	Mercaptopurine, Thioguanine	History of chronic hepatitis
Immune and spleen	Asplenia, Hyposplenia	Radiation ($\geq$40 Gy) impacting spleen, Splenectomy	History of chronic graft-versus-host disease
Nervous system	Peripheral sensory or motor neuropathy	Cisplatinincristine, Vinblastine vincristine	History of Charcot-Marie-Tooth disease
	Clinical leukoencephalopathy (spasticity, ataxia, dysarthria, dysphagia), Hemiparesis, Seizures	Methotrexate (high-dose intravenous or intrathecal), Cytarabine (high-dose intravenous or intrathecal), Radiation impacting the brain	Younger age at treatment at higher risk
Pulmonary	Interstitial pneumonitis, Pulmonary fibrosis, Restrictive lung disease, Obstructive lung disease	Bleomycin, Busulfan, Carmustine (BCNU), Lomustine (CCNU), Radiation impacting the lungs	Younger age at treatment at higher risk
Urinary tract: bladder	Hemorrhagic cystitis, Bladder fibrosis, Dysfunctional voiding, Vesicoureteral reflux, Hydronephrosis	Cyclophosphamide, Ifosfamide, Radiation impacting the bladder	No predisposing host factors
Urinary tract: kidney	Glomerular toxicity, Tubular toxicity (renal tubular acidosis, Fanconi's syndrome, hypophosphatemic rickets)	Cisplatin, Carboplatin, Ifosfamide, Radiation impacting the kidney	Mononephric
Vision	Cataracts	Busulfan, Radiation impacting the eye	No predisposing host factors

Table 3
Reproductive effects associated with childhood cancer

Reproductive effect	Predisposing therapy	Modifying host factors
Acute ovarian failure (ovarian failure within 5 y of diagnosis) Premature menopause (cessation of menses before age 40 y)	Alkylating agent chemotherapy Radiation impacting female reproductive system (whole abdomen, pelvis, lumbosacral spine, total body) Oophorectomy	Older age at treatment due at higher risk
Uterine vascular insufficiency	Radiation impacting the uterus (whole abdomen, pelvis, lumbosacral spine, total body)	History of Wilms' tumor and associated müllerian anomalies
Vaginal fibrosis or stenosis	Radiation impacting the vagina	History of hypogonadism (estrogen insufficiency) History of chronic graft-versus-host disease
Sexual dysfunction, dyspareunia, and so forth	Pelvic surgery, hysterectomy	History of hypogonadism (estrogen insufficiency) History of chronic graft-versus-host disease
Germ cell failure, oligospermia and azoospermia	Alkylating agent chemotherapy Radiation impacting the male reproductive system (pelvic, testicular, total body) Orchiectomy (bilateral)	Prepubertal status at treatment does not reduce risk
Retrograde ejaculation Anejaculation Erectile dysfunction	Pelvic surgery (retroperitoneal node dissection, dissectionretroperitoneal tumor resection, cystectomy, radical prostatectomy) Radiation to pelvis, bladder, or spine	History of hypogonadism (androgen insufficiency)
Adverse pregnancy outcomes Spontaneous abortion Neonatal death Low-birth-weight infant Fetal malposition Premature labor	Radiation impacting the uterus (whole abdomen, pelvis, lumbosacral spine, total body)	History of Wilms' tumor and associated müllerian anomalies

Table 4
Standardized incidence ratios of second and subsequent malignant neoplasms in the childhood cancer survivor study cohort

Second/subsequent malignancy	SIR (95% CI)	Median time to occurrence (y)
All second/subsequent malignancies	6.38 (5.69–7.13)	11.7
Acute myeloid leukemia	7.92 (3.61–15.04)	6.1
Lymphoma	1.51 (0.80–2.58)	13.8
Central nervous system tumor	9.85 (6.90–13.63)	9.5
Breast cancer	16.18 (12.35–20.83)	15.7
Bone cancer	19.14 (12.72–27.67)	9.6
Soft tissue sarcoma	6.33 (4.33–8.94)	10.6
Thyroid cancer	11.34 (8.20–15.27)	13.3
Melanoma	4.04 (2.43–6.32)	14.6
All other cancers	4.01 (3.05–5.18)	13.9

Abbreviations: CI, confidence intervals; SIR, standardized incidence ratio.
Data from Neglia JP, Friedman DL, Yasui Y, et al. Second malignant neoplasms in five-year survivors of childhood cancer: childhood cancer survivor study. J Natl Cancer Inst 2001;93:618–29.

2 to 3 years following topoisomerase II inhibitors. The risk of alkylating agent–associated leukemia increases with increasing cumulative dose, whereas the risk of topoisomerase inhibitor–related leukemia demonstrates both dose and schedule relationships. Radiation exposure has also been linked to an excess risk of secondary leukemia, but the magnitude of risk is much smaller [54]. The risk of radiation-related leukemia has been related to the radiation dose and volume of exposed active bone marrow. Because of cell killing at higher doses, the excess risk of leukemia per unit dose of radiation is greater at low versus high dose. Latency to onset is similar to that of alkylating agent–associated leukemia with a peak at 5 to 9 years after radiation. Secondary acute myeloid leukemia risk after these predisposing childhood cancer therapies plateaus after 10 years.

Radiation therapy predisposes to an excess risk of a variety of secondary solid tumors [45–51]. In contrast to secondary leukemia, the latency to onset of secondary solid tumors is much longer and typically exceeds 10 years without a demonstrable plateau. Secondary solid tumors in childhood cancer survivors most commonly involve the breast, thyroid, CNS, bones, and soft tissues [46,48,49,51]. With more prolonged follow-up of cohorts of adults surviving childhood cancer, epithelial neoplasms involving the gastrointestinal tract and lung have emerged [45,46]. Benign and low-grade malignancies including nonmelanoma skin cancer and meningiomas have also been observed with increasing prevalence in survivors treated with radiation for childhood cancer [47,49,50].

Data regarding the contribution of chemotherapy in solid tumor carcinogenesis in childhood cancer survivors are limited [55,56]. In studies of adults with lymphoma, secondary lung and bladder cancer risk exhibited a dose-dependent relationship with exposure to cytotoxic agents [57,58]. One pediatric cohort study observed that the risk of bone sarcomas increased in a linear fashion with increasing cumulative dose of alkylating agents [56]. Another recent study demonstrated that pediatric cancer patients concomitantly treated with chemoradiotherapy and radiation were significantly more at risk of developing a second cancer than were patients treated with sequential chemoradiotherapy [55]. The investigators did not observe a dose-effect relationship, however, between any drug category and the risk of a second cancer.

Breast cancer is the most common secondary solid tumor reported in childhood cancer survivors, with incidence rates ranging from 10% to 20% by 20 years from radiation [46,59–64]. Excess risk has been reported in female survivors treated with high-dose, extended-volume radiation at 30 years of age or younger [62]. Treatment with higher cumulative doses of alkylating agents and ovarian radiation greater than or equal to 5 Gy, exposures predisposing to premature menopause, have been correlated with reductions in breast cancer risk, underscoring the potential contribution of hormonal stimulation on breast carcinogenesis [63,65]. Because breast cancer risk begins to increase about 8 years after radiation, predisposed childhood cancer survivors are often younger than 40 years of age at diagnosis of breast cancer, the average age of breast cancer diagnoses in the general population. These data provide strong support for the implementation of breast cancer surveillance programs in these young at-risk women who would not routinely be participating in community breast cancer screening programs.

RISK-BASED CARE OF CHILDHOOD CANCER SURVIVORS

In pediatric oncology, investigations of health-related and quality-of-life outcomes in long-term survivors over the last 30 years have facilitated the identification of groups at high risk for morbidity based on host- or cancer-related factors. Knowledge gained from these studies has, in turn, informed strategies aiming to improve outcomes through primary interventions targeting newly diagnosed patients and secondary interventions focusing on long-term survivors determined to be predisposed to morbidity. Continuing this paradigm of care across the lifespan of the childhood cancer survivor provides opportunities to prevent or modify the risk and severity of many late effects. A wealth of data is available linking therapeutic exposures for childhood cancer to specific adverse outcomes that permits providers to anticipate cancer-related health risks. This risk-based care approach should include a systematic plan for lifelong screening, surveillance, and prevention that incorporates risks based on the previous cancer, cancer therapy, genetic predispositions, lifestyle behaviors, and comorbid health conditions [18,66]. Information critical to the coordination of risk-based care includes the date of cancer diagnosis; cancer histology; organs and tissues involved by cancer; and specific treatment modalities, such as surgical procedures, chemotherapeutic agents, and radiation treatment fields and doses; and history of bone marrow or stem cell transplant and blood product transfusion. Knowledge of cumulative dosages or dose intensity of chemotherapeutic agents like anthracycline or methotrexate is also important in estimating risk and determining screening frequency. Ideally, this information is organized in a treatment summary provided by the pediatric oncologist to the childhood cancer survivor and community providers. For survivors who have not been provided with this information, the Children's Oncology Group (COG) offers a template that can be used by survivors to organize a personal treatment summary (Fig. 1).

SUMMARY OF CANCER TREATMENT
(Comprehensive)

DEMOGRAPHICS				
Name: (last, first, middle)	**Sex:** (M/F)		**Date of Birth:**	**COG Reg #:**
Address: (number, street, city, state/province, postal code, country)				
Phone:	**SS#**		**Race/Ethnicity:**	
Alternate contact:		**Relationship:**		**Phone:**

CANCER DIAGNOSIS		
Diagnosis:		
Date of Diagnosis:	**Age at Diagnosis:**	**Date Therapy Completed:**
Sites involved/stage/diagnostic details:		**Laterality:** (Right/Left/NA)
Hereditary/congenital history:		
Pertinent past medical history:		
Treatment Center:		**Medical Record #:**
MD/APN Contact Information:		

RELAPSE(S) ☐ Yes ☐ No   *If yes, provide information below*

Date:	Site(s):	Laterality: (Right/Left/NA)	Date Therapy Completed:

SUBSEQUENT MALIGNANT NEOPLASM(S) ☐ Yes ☐ No   *If yes, provide information below*

Date:	Type:	
Stage/Site(s):		Date Therapy Completed:

CANCER TREATMENT SUMMARY

PROTOCOL(S) ☐ Yes ☐ No   *If yes, provide information below*

Acronym/Number	Title/Description	Initiated	Completed	On-Study

CHEMOTHERAPY ☐ Yes ☐ No   *If yes, complete chart below*

Drug Name	Route	Additional Information

* Anthracyclines: Include cumulative dose in mg/m^2; Carboplatin: Indicate if dose was myeloablative;
IV Methotrexate and Cytarabine: Indicate if any single dose was ≥1000 mg/m^2.
Note: Cumulative doses, if known, should be recorded for all agents, particularly for alkylators and bleomycin.

Fig. 1. Template form that can be used to develop a cancer treatment summary. (*Courtesy of* the Children's Oncology Group. Available at: www.survivorshipguidelines.org; with permission).

SUMMARY OF CANCER TREATMENT (continued)

RADIATION	☐ Yes	☐ No	*If yes, complete chart below*							
Site/Field	Laterality	Start Date	Stop Date	Fractions	Dose per Fraction (cGy)	Total Dose (cGy)	Boost Site	Boost Dose (cGy)	Total Dose with Boost (cGy)	Type

Radiation oncologist:		Institution:	

HEMATOPOIETIC CELL TRANSPLANT ☐ Yes ☐ No *If yes, complete chart below*				
Type	Source	Date of Infusion	Conditioning Regimen	Institution/Treating MD

Tandem? **Yes/No**

GVHD prophylaxis/treatment (For transplant patients only) ☐ Yes ☐ No *If yes, complete chart below*		
Type	First Dose	Last Dose

Was this patient ever diagnosed with **chronic** graft-versus-host disease (cGVHD)? ☐ Yes ☐ No

SURGERY ☐ Yes ☐ No *If yes, complete chart below*				
Date	Procedure	Site (if applicable)	Laterality (if applicable)	Surgeon/Institution

OTHER THERAPEUTIC MODALITIES ☐ Yes ☐ No *If yes, complete chart below*		
Therapy	Route	Cumulative Dose (if known)

COMPLICATIONS/LATE EFFECTS ☐ Yes ☐ No *If yes, complete chart below*			
Problem	Date onset	Date resolved	Status
			(Active/Resolved)
			(Active/Resolved)
			(Active/Resolved)
			(Active/Resolved)
			(Active/Resolved)
			(Active/Resolved)

Adverse Drug Reactions/Allergies ☐ Yes ☐ No *If yes, complete chart below*			
Drug	Reaction	Date	Status
			(Active/Resolved)
			(Active/Resolved)

Additional Information/Comments ☐ Yes ☐ No *If yes, provide information below*	

Summary prepared by: (name/title/institution)	Date prepared:
Summary updated by: (name/title/institution)	Date updated:

Fig. 1 *(continued)*

CHILDHOOD CANCER SURVIVOR CARE

Across the United States, there are many multidisciplinary long-term follow-up (LTFU) programs that work collaboratively with community physicians to provide care for childhood cancer survivors. This type of shared care has been proposed as the optimal model to facilitate coordination between the cancer center oncology team and community physician groups providing survivor care [67]. Where available, childhood cancer survivors maintaining remission are transitioned from the treating oncology team to a LTFU program 2 or more years after completion of therapy. Comprehensive LTFU programs provide multidisciplinary care at a specified time and place that is typically directed by a pediatric oncologist or other subspecialist and coordinated by an oncology nurse or nurse practitioner [68]. Standard services offered by comprehensive LTFU programs include risk-based health screening; referral to appropriate specialists; and education regarding cancer history, cancer-related health risks, and prevention and risk reduction measures to maintain wellness. Only rarely are survivors permitted to continue follow-up in pediatric LTFU programs during adulthood; however, transition programs are available at a limited number of centers for older survivors who can no longer be monitored at pediatric institutions.

In general, most survivors in the United States eventually return to community providers for their primary and cancer-related care. An essential service of LTFU programs is to facilitate the transition from oncology to community care by organizing an individualized survivorship care plan that includes details about therapeutic interventions undertaken for childhood cancer and their potential health risks, personalized health screening recommendations, and information about lifestyle factors that modify risks. The survivorship prescription is extremely important because the survivor's contact with the cancer center becomes less frequent with increasing passage of time from diagnosis and therapy [69]. Community physicians are then challenged with providing care for survivors who often lack knowledge about specific details of their cancer history [70].

The relative rarity of childhood cancer, its heterogeneous histologic subtypes, and the diverse and evolving treatment approaches used over the years offer limited opportunity or incentive for community physicians to increase their expertise in survivor care. These data suggest that survivor care is optimally delivered in specialty clinics that are staffed by clinicians familiar with long-term health risks associated with childhood cancer. These comprehensive LTFU programs are limited in number, however, and frequently struggle with solvency [68]. System-driven barriers to the functioning of these programs include lack of adequate resources and financial support, low institutional commitment to survivorship care, limited capacity for survivor care, and difficulty in communication with community physicians [68]. Survivor-driven barriers to success of LTFU programs include lack of interest or awareness about health risks associated with cancer. Finally, for many survivors who appreciate the need for late effects monitoring after cancer, LTFU programs are not available to all survivors because of financial or geographic reasons or because they are too old to continue care in the pediatric cancer center. Collectively, these data support the need for interventions that facilitate risk-based survivor care in the community setting.

GUIDELINES FOR FOLLOW-UP CARE AFTER CHILDHOOD CANCER

Recognizing that most survivors do not have access to late effects experts in their community to coordinate health care after cancer, many pediatric cancer centers have focused on patient education and self-advocacy as a means of disseminating awareness about cancer-related health risks to community providers [71]. The availability of resources with reliable and succinct information about cancer-related late effects can enhance these efforts that target busy clinicians who are typically unfamiliar with unique health risks of the childhood cancer survivor. To address this need, several groups have developed health screening guidelines aiming to facilitate and standardize risk-based care of childhood cancer survivors [72–74]. Despite the abundant literature published about health outcomes after pediatric cancer, efforts to mount an evidence-base to support specific screening recommendations proved to be challenging for these groups for several reasons. (1) Evidence linking therapeutic exposures to specific adverse outcomes is limited by the lack of standard definitions of toxicity, use of variable testing strategies, and inconsistency in evaluation time in relation to exposure. (2) Many treatment effects are delayed in onset from the time of exposure. Comprehensive ascertainment of health outcomes in predisposed survivor groups becomes more difficult after pediatric survivors leave the cancer center. (3) A considerable number of late effects studies evaluate cohorts of convenience and are potentially biased because of incomplete participation of the at-risk cohort. (4) Because childhood cancer comprises a relatively small proportion of cancer diagnoses, establishing through randomized clinical trials that screening of asymptomatic survivors can reduce morbidity and mortality is not feasible. Consequently, studies evaluating usefulness and cost-effectiveness of screening asymptomatic survivors are unlikely to be undertaken.

Notwithstanding this imperfect evidence base, the imminent need of the medically vulnerable and growing population of childhood cancer survivors prompted the use of a hybrid-model for the development of health screening recommendations. Group methods varied in the magnitude and scope of the literature review, which provided evidence linking late effects with therapeutic exposures. All proposed screening recommendations, however, are based on the clinical experience of late effects experts matching the magnitude of the risk with the intensity of the screening recommendations. A brief description of the guideline development methodology undertaken by the COG, the Scottish Intercollegiate Guideline Network (SIGN), and the Late Effects Group of the United Kingdom Children's Cancer Study Group (UKCCSG) follows.

The Children's Oncology Group Guidelines

The COG Late Effects and Nursing Committee released Version 1.0 of the COG Guidelines to the COG membership in March 2003 [75]. This is a therapy-based design to permit modular formatting by therapeutic exposure and based on the patient's age, presenting features, and treatment era. The screening recommendations outlined in the COG Guidelines are appropriate for asymptomatic survivors presenting for routine exposure-based medical follow-up 2 or more years after completion of therapy for a childhood, adolescent, or young adult cancer. More extensive evaluations are presumed, as clinically indicated, for survivors presenting with signs and symptoms suggesting illness or organ dysfunction. Patient education materials called "Health Links" provide detailed information on guideline-specific topics to enhance health maintenance and promotion among this population of cancer survivors.

A multidisciplinary panel of late effects experts scored the Guidelines according to a modified version of the National Comprehensive Cancer Network "Categories of Consensus" system [76]. Each score reflects the expert panel's assessment of the strength of evidence from the literature linking specific adverse outcomes to specific therapeutic exposures during childhood cancer coupled with an assessment of the appropriateness of the screening recommendation based on the expert panel's collective clinical experience. "High-level evidence" was defined as evidence derived from high-quality case control or cohort studies. "Lower-level evidence" was defined as evidence derived from nonanalytic studies, case reports, case series, and clinical experience. All "Category 1" recommendations reflect uniform consensus among the reviewers. "Category 2" recommendations are designated as "2A" (there is uniformity of consensus among the reviewers regarding strength of evidence and appropriateness of the screening recommendation) or "2B" (there is nonuniform consensus among the reviewers regarding strength of evidence and appropriateness of the screening recommendation). Rather than submitting recommendations representing major disagreements, items scored as "Category 3" were either deleted or revised by the panel of experts to provide at least a "Category 2B" score for all recommendations included in the guidelines.

Multidisciplinary system-based (eg, cardiovascular, neurocognitive, reproductive, and so forth) task forces organized within the COG Late Effects Committee are responsible for monitoring the literature, evaluating guideline content, and providing recommendations for guideline revision as new information becomes available. The task forces' efforts have prompted several revisions of the COG Guidelines to ensure consistency with survivor health outcomes reported in the literature. The currently available COG Guidelines Version 2.0 features 136 sections detailing exposure-based potential late effects and health screening recommendations, cancer screening recommendations for standard and high-risk groups, and 42 "Health Links." COG Guidelines Version 3.0 is scheduled for release in the spring of 2008. The COG Guidelines and their accompanying health education materials are available at: http://www.survivorshipguidelines.org.

The Scottish Intercollegiate Guideline Network Guidelines

The SIGN published national guidelines for pediatric cancer survivors, Long Term Follow Up of Survivors of Childhood Cancer - SIGN 76, in January 2004 and updated these recommendations in March 2005 [72]. The SIGN guidelines represent the results of a systematic review and critical appraisal of the literature [77]. At least two independent reviewers evaluated eligible studies and rated their methodologic quality as low-risk of bias (all or most methodologic criteria met) or high-risk of bias (few or no criteria fulfilled) with corresponding scores ranging from "1++" to "4." A multidisciplinary review team, based on their collective clinical experience and knowledge of the evidence, assigned graded recommendations for use in guiding management decisions. Grades range from "A" to "D," with an "A" representing the highest level of evidence available (eg, randomized clinical trials with very low risk of bias), and "D" representing evidence extrapolated from nonanalytic studies or expert opinion. Recommended best practices, based on the clinical experience of the guideline development group, are indicated by a check mark.

The SIGN Guidelines provide a in-depth analysis of five key survivor outcomes, along with rationale for the assigned grading of each recommendation: (1) assessment and achievement of normal growth; (2) achievement of normal progression through puberty and factors affecting fertility; (3) early identification, assessment, and treatment of cardiac abnormalities; (4) assessment of thyroid function; and (5) assessment and achievement of optimum neurodevelopment and psychologic health. In addition to clinical recommendations, the SIGN guideline contains recommendations for delivery of LTFU care for pediatric cancer survivors based on the intensity of treatment received [78]. The degree of long-term risk is determined by site of the underlying malignancy, type and intensity of treatment, and patient age at treatment. The recommended levels of follow-up are summarized in Table 5. The entire SIGN guideline is available at: http://www.sign.ac.uk/guidelines/fulltext/76.

The United Kingdom Children's Cancer Study Group Practice Statement

In 1995, the UKCCSG Late Effects Group released the first edition of Practice Statement "Therapy Based Long Term Follow Up" [73]. The purpose of the Practice Statement is to inform and guide clinicians responsible for the clinical follow-up of long-term childhood cancer survivors. The Practice Statement

Table 5
Scottish Intercollegiate Guideline Network recommended levels of long-term follow-up of childhood cancer survivors

Level	Method of long-term follow-up	Frequency of long-term follow-up	Treatment	Examples
1	Mail or telephone	Every 1–2 y	Surgery alone Low-risk chemotherapy	Wilms' tumor, stage I or II, germ cell tumors (surgery only)
2	Led by nurse or primary care doctor	Every 1–2 y	Chemotherapy Low-dose (≤24 Gy) cranial radiotherapy	Most patients (eg, acute lymphoblastic leukemia in first remission)
3	Medically supervised long-term follow-up clinic	Annual	Radiotherapy (except low-dose cranial radiotherapy)	Brain tumors After bone marrow transplantation Any stage IV tumor

Appropriate for childhood cancer survivors more than 5 years after completion of therapy.
Adapted from Wallace WH, Blacklay A, Eiser C, et al. Developing strategies for long term follow up of survivors of childhood cancer. BMJ 2001;323:271–4; with permission.

provides recommendations regarding the content of LTFU including clinical assessment by medical history, physical examination, diagnostic investigations, and suggestions for further follow-up. The document includes a brief summary of exposure-based (any treatment, chemotherapy, radiation, surgery) outcomes followed by 25 key content sections highlighting potential adverse outcomes related to childhood cancer. In addition, nine appendices elaborate further detail about health outcomes in high-risk populations (survivors of CNS tumors or hematopoietic cell transplant) or issues of broad importance across diagnostic types (puberty, infertility, immunization). The content is presented in a user-friendly format targeting professional end users, such as nurses working in LTFU clinics. A second edition of the Practice Statement was updated in June 2006 and is available at: http://www.ukccsg.org/public/followup/PracticeStatement.

Benefits and Limitations of Guidelines

The recommendations outlined in the COG and SIGN Guidelines and UKCCSG Practice Statement offer survivors the potential benefits of early identification of and intervention for late-onset therapy-related complications. Survivors may also experience potential harms, however, including anxiety related to increased awareness of health risks and false-positive screening evaluations. In addition, the costs of LTFU care may be prohibitive for some patients. Benefits and harms are particularly pertinent to consider because evidence supporting optimal screening methods for many outcomes and the benefits of treating asymptomatic survivors with subclinical dysfunction have not been established. Collectively, these data underscore the need for prospective research to identify effective screening modalities and appropriate screening frequency and to establish the impact of screening on long-term survivor health outcomes.

SUMMARY

Following treatment for childhood cancer, late health effects are common and become more prevalent with increasing passage of time after completion of therapy. Because of extensive research linking therapeutic exposures with specific treatment complications, many late effects can be anticipated and proactively addressed to reduce cancer-related morbidity. Providers should be aware of health screening guideline resources that can be used to facilitate survivor care. Because many late effects of childhood cancer manifest during adulthood after the survivor has been transitioned to the care of community physicians, coordination of an individualized survivorship care plan between oncology and community providers is essential to optimize long-term risk-based survivor care.

References

[1] Ries LAG, Harkins D, Krapcho M, et al. SEER Cancer Statistics Review, 1975–2003. Available at: http://seer.cancer.gov/csr/1975_2003.
[2] Hewitt M, Weiner SL, Simone JV, editors. Childhood cancer survivorship: improving care and quality of life. Washington, DC: National Cancer Policy Board; 2003.

[3] Jemal A, Siegel R, Ward E, et al. Cancer statistics, 2006. CA Cancer J Clin 2006;56: 106–30.

[4] Geenen MM, Cardous-Ubbink MC, Kremer LC, et al. Medical assessment of adverse health outcomes in long-term survivors of childhood cancer. JAMA 2007;297:2705–15.

[5] Oeffinger KC, Mertens AC, Sklar CA, et al. Chronic health conditions in adult survivors of childhood cancer. N Engl J Med 2006;355:1572–82.

[6] Bhatia S, Francisco L, Carter A, et al. Late mortality after allogeneic hematopoietic cell transplantation and functional status of long-term survivors: report from the Bone Marrow Transplant Survivor Study. Blood 2007;110:3784–92.

[7] Hudson MM, Mertens AC, Yasui Y, et al. Health status of adult long-term survivors of childhood cancer: a report from the Childhood Cancer Survivor Study. JAMA 2003;290: 1583–92.

[8] Ness KK, Mertens AC, Hudson MM, et al. Limitations on physical performance and daily activities among long-term survivors of childhood cancer. Ann Intern Med 2005;143: 639–47.

[9] Ness KK, Wall MM, Oakes JM, et al. Physical performance limitations and participation restrictions among cancer survivors: a population-based study. Ann Epidemiol 2006;16: 197–205.

[10] Schultz KA, Ness KK, Whitton J, et al. Behavioral and social outcomes in adolescent survivors of childhood cancer: a report from the childhood cancer survivor study. J Clin Oncol 2007;25:3649–56.

[11] Speechley KN, Barrera M, Shaw AK, et al. Health-related quality of life among child and adolescent survivors of childhood cancer. J Clin Oncol 2006;24:2536–43.

[12] Zebrack BJ, Gurney JG, Oeffinger K, et al. Psychological outcomes in long-term survivors of childhood brain cancer: a report from the childhood cancer survivor study. J Clin Oncol 2004;22:999–1006.

[13] Zebrack BJ, Zeltzer LK, Whitton J, et al. Psychological outcomes in long-term survivors of childhood leukemia, Hodgkin's disease, and non-Hodgkin's lymphoma: a report from the Childhood Cancer Survivor Study. Pediatrics 2002;110:42–52.

[14] Zebrack BJ, Zevon MA, Turk N, et al. Psychological distress in long-term survivors of solid tumors diagnosed in childhood: a report from the childhood cancer survivor study. Pediatr Blood Cancer 2007;49:47–51.

[15] Mertens AC. Cause of mortality in 5-year survivors of childhood cancer. Pediatr Blood Cancer 2007;48:723–6.

[16] Bhatia S, Meadows AT. Long-term follow-up of childhood cancer survivors: future directions for clinical care and research. Pediatr Blood Cancer 2006;46:143–8.

[17] Alvarez JA, Scully RE, Miller TL, et al. Long-term effects of treatments for childhood cancers. Curr Opin Pediatr 2007;19:23–31.

[18] Oeffinger KC, Hudson MM. Long-term complications following childhood and adolescent cancer: foundations for providing risk-based health care for survivors. CA Cancer J Clin 2004;54:208–36.

[19] Fletcher BD. Effects of pediatric cancer therapy on the musculoskeletal system. Pediatr Radiol 1997;27:623–36.

[20] Nunez SB, Mulrooney DA, Laverdiere C, et al. Risk-based health monitoring of childhood cancer survivors: a report from the children's oncology group. Curr Oncol Rep 2007;9: 440–52.

[21] Rutter MM, Rose SR. Long-term endocrine sequelae of childhood cancer. Curr Opin Pediatr 2007;19:480–7.

[22] Sala A, Mattano LA Jr, Barr RD. Osteonecrosis in children and adolescents with cancer: an adverse effect of systemic therapy. Eur J Cancer 2007;43:683–9.

[23] Sala A, Barr RD. Osteopenia and cancer in children and adolescents: the fragility of success. Cancer 2007;109:1420–31.

[24] Armstrong GT, Sklar CA, Hudson MM, et al. Long-term health status among survivors of childhood cancer: does sex matter? J Clin Oncol 2007;25:4477–89.

[25] Butler RW, Haser JK. Neurocognitive effects of treatment for childhood cancer. Ment Retard Dev Disabil Res Rev 2006;12:184–91.

[26] Barry E, Alvarez JA, Scully RE, et al. Anthracycline-induced cardiotoxicity: course, pathophysiology, prevention and management. Expert Opin Pharmacother 2007;8:1039–58.

[27] Lipshultz SE, Lipsitz SR, Sallan SE, et al. Chronic progressive cardiac dysfunction years after doxorubicin therapy for childhood acute lymphoblastic leukemia. J Clin Oncol 2005;23: 2629–36.

[28] Gower WA, Collaco JM, Mogayzel PJ Jr. Pulmonary dysfunction in pediatric hematopoietic stem cell transplant patients: non-infectious and long-term complications. Pediatr Blood Cancer 2007;49:225–33.

[29] Stohr W, Paulides M, Bielack S, et al. Nephrotoxicity of cisplatin and carboplatin in sarcoma patients: a report from the late effects surveillance system. Pediatr Blood Cancer 2007;48:140–7.

[30] Stohr W, Paulides M, Bielack S, et al. Ifosfamide-induced nephrotoxicity in 593 sarcoma patients: a report from the Late Effects Surveillance System. Pediatr Blood Cancer 2007;48:447–52.

[31] Abramson DH, Beaverson KL, Chang ST, et al. Outcome following initial external beam radiotherapy in patients with Reese-Ellsworth group Vb retinoblastoma. Arch Ophthalmol 2004;122:1316–23.

[32] Knight KR, Kraemer DF, Neuwelt EA. Ototoxicity in children receiving platinum chemotherapy: underestimating a commonly occurring toxicity that may influence academic and social development. J Clin Oncol 2005;23:8588–96.

[33] Jacobsen KD, Ous S, Waehre H, et al. Ejaculation in testicular cancer patients after post-chemotherapy retroperitoneal lymph node dissection. Br J Cancer 1999;80:249–55.

[34] Spunt SL, Sweeney TA, Hudson MM, et al. Late effects of pelvic rhabdomyosarcoma and its treatment in female survivors. J Clin Oncol 2005;23:7143–51.

[35] Muller J. Impact of cancer therapy on the reproductive axis. Horm Res 2003;1(Suppl 59): 12–20.

[36] Thomson AB, Critchley HO, Kelnar CJ, et al. Late reproductive sequelae following treatment of childhood cancer and options for fertility preservation. Best Pract Res Clin Endocrinol Metab 2002;16:311–34.

[37] Chemaitilly W, Mertens AC, Mitby P, et al. Acute ovarian failure in the childhood cancer survivor study. J Clin Endocrinol Metab 2006;91:1723–8.

[38] Sklar CA, Mertens AC, Mitby P, et al. Premature menopause in survivors of childhood cancer: a report from the childhood cancer survivor study. J Natl Cancer Inst 2006;98:890–6.

[39] Bath LE, Wallace WH, Critchley HO. Late effects of the treatment of childhood cancer on the female reproductive system and the potential for fertility preservation. BJOG 2002;109: 107–14.

[40] Critchley HO, Bath LE, Wallace WH. Radiation damage to the uterus: review of the effects of treatment of childhood cancer. Hum Fertil (Camb) 2002;5:61–6.

[41] Kenney LB, Nicholson HS, Brasseux C, et al. Birth defects in offspring of adult survivors of childhood acute lymphoblastic leukemia. A Childrens Cancer Group/National Institutes of Health Report. Cancer 1996;78:169–76.

[42] Nagarajan R, Robison LL. Pregnancy outcomes in survivors of childhood cancer. J Natl Cancer Inst Monogr 2005;34:72–6.

[43] Signorello LB, Cohen SS, Bosetti C, et al. Female survivors of childhood cancer: preterm birth and low birth weight among their children. J Natl Cancer Inst 2006;98:1453–61.

[44] Travis LB, Rabkin CS, Brown LM, et al. Cancer survivorship–genetic susceptibility and second primary cancers: research strategies and recommendations. J Natl Cancer Inst 2006;98:15–25.

[45] Bassal M, Mertens AC, Taylor L, et al. Risk of selected subsequent carcinomas in survivors of childhood cancer: a report from the Childhood Cancer Survivor Study. J Clin Oncol 2006;24:476–83.

[46] Bhatia S, Yasui Y, Robison LL, et al. High risk of subsequent neoplasms continues with extended follow-up of childhood Hodgkin's disease: report from the Late Effects Study Group. J Clin Oncol 2003;21:4386–94.

[47] Hijiya N, Hudson MM, Lensing S, et al. Cumulative incidence of secondary neoplasms as a first event after childhood acute lymphoblastic leukemia. JAMA 2007;297:1207–15.

[48] Neglia JP, Friedman DL, Yasui Y, et al. Second malignant neoplasms in five-year survivors of childhood cancer: childhood cancer survivor study. J Natl Cancer Inst 2001;93:618–29.

[49] Neglia JP, Robison LL, Stovall M, et al. New primary neoplasms of the central nervous system in survivors of childhood cancer: a report from the Childhood Cancer Survivor Study. J Natl Cancer Inst 2006;98:1528–37.

[50] Perkins JL, Liu Y, Mitby PA, et al. Nonmelanoma skin cancer in survivors of childhood and adolescent cancer: a report from the childhood cancer survivor study. J Clin Oncol 2005;23:3733–41.

[51] Ronckers CM, Sigurdson AJ, Stovall M, et al. Thyroid cancer in childhood cancer survivors: a detailed evaluation of radiation dose response and its modifiers. Radiat Res 2006;166: 618–28.

[52] Meadows AT, Obringer AC, Marrero O, et al. Second malignant neoplasms following childhood Hodgkin's disease: treatment and splenectomy as risk factors. Med Pediatr Oncol 1989;17:477–84.

[53] Smith MA, Rubinstein L, Anderson JR, et al. Secondary leukemia or myelodysplastic syndrome after treatment with epipodophyllotoxins. J Clin Oncol 1999;17:569–77.

[54] Van Leeuwen FE, Travis LB. Second cancers. In: DeVita VT, Hellman S, Rosenberg SA, editors. Cancer: principles and practice of oncology. 7th edition. Philadelphia: Lippincott Williams and Wilkins; 2005. p. 2575–602.

[55] Guerin S, Guibout C, Shamsaldin A, et al. Concomitant chemo-radiotherapy and local dose of radiation as risk factors for second malignant neoplasms after solid cancer in childhood: a case-control study. Int J Cancer 2007;120:96–102.

[56] Hawkins MM, Wilson LM, Burton HS, et al. Radiotherapy, alkylating agents, and risk of bone cancer after childhood cancer. J Natl Cancer Inst 1996;88:270–8.

[57] Travis LB, Curtis RE, Glimelius B, et al. Bladder and kidney cancer following cyclophosphamide therapy for non-Hodgkin's lymphoma. J Natl Cancer Inst 1995;87:524–30.

[58] Travis LB, Gilbert E. Lung cancer after Hodgkin lymphoma: the roles of chemotherapy, radiotherapy and tobacco use. Radiat Res 2005;163:695–6.

[59] Dores GM, Metayer C, Curtis RE, et al. Second malignant neoplasms among long-term survivors of Hodgkin's disease: a population-based evaluation over 25 years. J Clin Oncol 2002;20:3484–94.

[60] Kenney LB, Yasui Y, Inskip PD, et al. Breast cancer after childhood cancer: a report from the Childhood Cancer Survivor Study. Ann Intern Med 2004;141:590–7.

[61] Metayer C, Lynch CF, Clarke EA, et al. Second cancers among long-term survivors of Hodgkin's disease diagnosed in childhood and adolescence. J Clin Oncol 2000;18:2435–43.

[62] Travis LB, Hill D, Dores GM, et al. Cumulative absolute breast cancer risk for young women treated for Hodgkin lymphoma. J Natl Cancer Inst 2005;97:1428–37.

[63] Travis LB, Hill DA, Dores GM, et al. Breast cancer following radiotherapy and chemotherapy among young women with Hodgkin disease. JAMA 2003;290:465–75.

[64] van Leeuwen FE, Klokman WJ, Veer MB, et al. Long-term risk of second malignancy in survivors of Hodgkin's disease treated during adolescence or young adulthood. J Clin Oncol 2000;18:487–97.

[65] van Leeuwen FE, Klokman WJ, Stovall M, et al. Roles of radiation dose, chemotherapy, and hormonal factors in breast cancer following Hodgkin's disease. J Natl Cancer Inst 2003;95: 971–80.

[66] Oeffinger KC. Longitudinal risk-based health care for adult survivors of childhood cancer. Curr Probl Cancer 2003;27:143–67.

[67] Oeffinger KC, McCabe MS. Models for delivering survivorship care. J Clin Oncol 2006;24: 5117–24.

[68] Aziz NM, Oeffinger KC, Brooks S, et al. Comprehensive long-term follow-up programs for pediatric cancer survivors. Cancer 2006;107:841–8.

[69] Oeffinger KC, Mertens AC, Hudson MM, et al. Health care of young adult survivors of childhood cancer: a report from the Childhood Cancer Survivor Study. Ann Fam Med 2004;2:61–70.

[70] Kadan-Lottick NS, Robison LL, Gurney JG, et al. Childhood cancer survivors' knowledge about their past diagnosis and treatment: Childhood Cancer Survivor Study. JAMA 2002;287:1832–9.

[71] Landier W, Wallace WH, Hudson MM. Long-term follow-up of pediatric cancer survivors: education, surveillance, and screening. Pediatr Blood Cancer 2006;46:149–58.

[72] Long term follow up of survivors of childhood cancer. Guideline no. 76. Available at: http://www.sign.ac.uk/pdf/sign76.pdf.

[73] Therapy based long-term follow up: practice statement. United Kingdom Children's Cancer Study Group Late Effects Group. Available at: http://www.ukccsg.org/public/followup/PracticeStatement/index.html.

[74] Long-term follow-up guidelines for survivors of childhood, adolescent and young adult cancer. March 2006; Version 2.0. Available at: http://www.survivorshipguidelines.org.

[75] Landier W, Bhatia S, Eshelman DA, et al. Development of risk-based guidelines for pediatric cancer survivors: the children's oncology group long-term follow-up guidelines from the children's oncology group late effects committee and nursing discipline. J Clin Oncol 2004;22: 4979–90.

[76] Winn RJ, Botnick WZ. The NCCN Guideline Program: a conceptual framework. Oncology (Williston Park) 1997;11:25–32.

[77] SIGN 50-A guideline developers handbook. Available at: http://www.sign.ac.uk/guidelines/fulltext/50/index.html.

[78] Wallace WH, Blacklay A, Eiser C, et al. Developing strategies for long term follow up of survivors of childhood cancer. BMJ 2001;323:271–4.

Hodgkin Lymphoma: The Follow-Up of Long-Term Survivors

David C. Hodgson, MD, MPH

Department of Radiation Oncology, University of Toronto, Princess Margaret Hospital, 610 University Avenue, Toronto M5G 2M9, Canada

Hodgkin lymphoma (HL) is a disease that typically strikes children and young adults, with more than 80% of those affected being cured [1–3]. Consequently, HL survivors can live for decades with the persistent and late-emerging effects of the disease and its treatment. These survivors are at increased risk for various health problems, including second cancers (SCs), heart disease, hormonal dysfunction, and infertility, and it is increasingly apparent that they require health care specifically tailored to take these risks into consideration. Several panels of clinical experts have issued guidelines to assist physicians in the long-term medical management of cancer survivors in general, and HL survivors in particular [4–8]. The focus of this article is the long-term medical management of HL survivors, specifically those who are 5 years or more off therapy without evidence of relapse, when the focus of follow-up care shifts from detecting relapse to minimizing the morbidity associated with the late effects of treatment.

SCREENING FOR SECOND CANCERS

SCs are a leading cause of morbidity and death among long-term survivors of HL [9–11]. Most SCs are solid tumors and typically occur after a minimal latency of 5 to 10 years, with breast cancers and lung cancers accounting for the largest absolute excess risk [10]. Risk factors for breast cancer among female HL survivors include young age at mediastinal radiation therapy (RT) (ie, age <30 years) and increasing dose of radiation, whereas patients who have experienced premature menopause because of treatment are at lesser risk [12]. Risk factors for lung cancer include chest irradiation (dose-related), alkylating agent chemotherapy (dose-related), and smoking (which has a supra-additive effect with treatment exposure) [13,14].

Breast Cancer Screening and Prevention

Clinical practice guidelines recommend the early initiation of breast cancer screening among female HL survivors who have had mediastinal RT [15].

E-mail address: david.hodgson@rmp.uhn.on.ca

0889-8588/08/$ – see front matter
doi:10.1016/j.hoc.2008.01.004

An important consideration is that the relatively high density of breast tissue in some young women may reduce the sensitivity of mammographic screening. Although some studies have found that most breast cancers in HL survivors are identifiable on mammograms, others have found that among female survivors undergoing mammographic surveillance, approximately 50% of breast cancers are detected clinically as palpable masses and many have adverse pathologic features (Table 1) [16,17]. This finding suggests that mammography alone may not provide optimal breast cancer screening in young female HL survivors.

The UK Royal College of Radiology recommends the initiation of breast cancer screening 8 years after mediastinal RT, or age 25, whichever is later [15]. Annual bilateral breast MRI is recommended for those younger than 30 years of age, whereas mammography is recommended for those aged 50 years or older. For women aged 30 to 49, initial mammography is recommended with this modality continued alone for those who have adequate mammographic quality. For those who have mammographically dense breast tissue, annual MRI is recommended in addition to mammography. For these patients, mammography is used to detect microcalcifications of ductal carcinoma in situ, which may be missed on MRI. In view of the evidence that screened women can still develop palpable tumors between annual mammography, women should also be encouraged to perform monthly self–breast examination and have yearly breast examination by a health care professional.

Ideally, a primary prevention strategy could be used to reduce the incidence of second breast cancers in these survivors. One study using a Markov model to estimate the effect of tamoxifen chemoprevention on the risk for breast cancer death in young women following mantle RT predicted that this intervention would produce significant improvement in survival and was cost effective [18]. A feasibility study was able to enroll only 11.5% of eligible patients, however, largely because of concerns about the side effects of tamoxifen [19]. Currently, chemoprevention strategies to reduce breast cancer risk in these survivors are investigational.

Lung Cancer Screening and Prevention

The benefit of screening for lung cancer with low-dose CT remains unknown, and several prospective trials are evaluating this intervention among high-risk

Table 1
Summary of breast cancer detection with mammographic screening of female Hodgkin lymphoma survivors

Author	Screened patients	Cancers detected			Detected by mammogram only	Clinically palpable	Node positive
		Total	Invasive	DCIS			
Diller et al, [17]	79	12	10	2	7 (58%)	5 (42%)	2 (17%)
Lee et al, [16]	100	12	7	5	5 (42%)	7 (58%)	6 (50%)

Abbreviation: DCIS, ductal carcinoma in situ.

patients (ie, smokers) in the general population [20,21]. The results of these studies do not easily generalize to HL survivors, however, many of whom have exposure to radiation and alkylating chemotherapy agents that increase the risk for lung cancer. A decision analysis evaluating annual low-dose CT screening in patients 5 years or more after mediastinal RT predicted it to be cost effective, particularly among smokers, with a survival gain comparable to other well-accepted cancer screening strategies [22]. An important consideration is that the absolute risk for lung cancer differs significantly among different groups of HL survivors. Nonsmoking patients treated before age 40 with contemporary chemotherapy (eg, doxorubicin, bleomycin, vinblastine, dacarbazine; ABVD) have a low absolute risk for lung cancer and it is unlikely that they would benefit from screening. Risk is highest among those treated with chest RT and alkylator-based chemotherapy at ages older than 40 years, particularly if they are smokers. Prospective trials of CT screening have been proposed to identify which survivors are likely to benefit; currently, CT screening remains investigational and is not widely used in routine practice. Routine chest radiographs have not been found to be an effective means of screening for lung cancer among smokers and are unlikely to be useful among long-term HL survivors.

Most individuals are aware that smoking increases their risk for lung cancer. Survivors often do not appreciate that smoking may increase their lung cancer risk significantly more than it does for the friends or family with whom they share the activity, however, and they may be unaware of the dismal prognosis associated with a lung cancer diagnosis. When relevant, survivors who smoke should be made aware that their prior exposure to mediastinal RT or alkylating agents enhances the smoking-related damage to their lungs. Physicians should not underestimate their own influence on a survivor's ability to quit; even brief advice on smoking cessation during an office visit has been shown to improve success rates. Pharmacotherapy improves the probability of success, and should be considered when there are no medical contraindications. There are several resources to assist physicians in the treatment of nicotine addiction [23].

Screening for Other Cancers

HL survivors may be at increased risk for several other forms of cancer in addition to lung and breast cancer. The risk for cervix cancer seems to be increased and female HL survivors should undergo cervix cancer screening according to established guidelines for the general population. Currently there is no evidence that increasing the frequency of screening in this population is necessary.

Colorectal cancer (CRC) risk is elevated among HL survivors. North American clinical practice guidelines recommend that people of average CRC risk in the general population should start screening at 50 years of age [24,25]. Notably, the risk for CRC in HL survivors is comparable to that of an average 50-year-old at a significantly younger age (Fig. 1), and some expert groups suggest that CRC screening be considered before age 50 for selected survivors. For example, the Children's Oncology Group (COG) recommends early CRC screening among patients who have undergone pelvic or abdominal

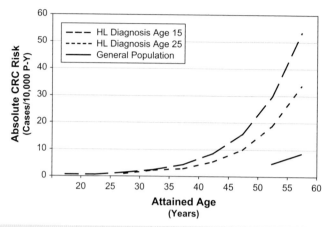

Fig. 1. Increased absolute risk for colorectal cancer (CRC) in HL survivors. North American practice guidelines generally recommend that CRC screening be initiated in the average risk population starting at age 50, when the absolute risk is approximately 5–10/10,000 person-years (*solid line*). HL survivors treated at age 15 or 25 experience this degree of risk starting at approximately age 40, several years before screening would otherwise be recommended. (*Data from* Hodgson DC, Gilbert ES, Dores GM, et al. Long-term solid cancer risk among 5-year survivors of Hodgkin's lymphoma. J Clin Oncol 2007;25(12):1489–97.)

RT to doses greater than 25 Gy, to be started 15 years after treatment or at age 35, whichever comes later [7]. Several forms of screening (eg, evaluation of fecal occult blood with or without sigmoidoscopy; colonoscopy) are appropriate and the US Preventive Services Taskforce (USPSTF) concluded that there were no persuasive data to support one form of screening over another in the general population.

Evaluation of Symptoms

In some circumstances, appreciation of the increased risk for SC among HL survivors should change how clinical symptoms are evaluated. Common problems, such as persistent cough or bony pains, may warrant more aggressive imaging evaluation to rule out malignancy in an HL survivor than might otherwise be undertaken in a young patient, particularly, for example, if persistent pain arises in a previously irradiated site. Similarly, thyroid cancer risk is elevated in HL survivors treated with neck RT. Thyroid nodules of any size in such a patient should be evaluated with ultrasound-guided fine needle aspiration, with surgical removal in the case of indeterminate or nondiagnostic results [26].

SCREENING AND PREVENTION OF CARDIOVASCULAR DISEASE

The risk for heart disease is significantly increased among HL survivors 5 to 10 years after treatment, and seems to increase with time [27,28]. Coronary artery disease accounts for most of the risk, although other cardiac problems may also arise, including valvular disease, pericardial disease, ventricular dysfunction, and conduction abnormalities. Mediastinal RT and doxorubicin-based chemotherapy are the main treatment-related risk factors.

A significant proportion of the excess risk occurs among survivors who have other cardiac risk factors [28]. HL survivors should be screened every 2 to 3 years for hypertension, hypercholesterolemia, and diabetes mellitus, and treated according to existing guidelines if these develop. Smokers should engage in a smoking cessation program. In addition, survivors should be encouraged to engage in regular exercise and maintain appropriate body weight.

Ventricular Dysfunction

Survivors treated as children with anthracyclines or mediastinal RT are at increased risk for delayed ventricular dysfunction. A review of 25 studies found subclinical cardiotoxicity in up to 57% of pediatric cancer survivors treated with 45 to 1275 mg/m^2 of anthracycline [29]. Although it is clear that subclinical cardiac dysfunction can be identified in these survivors, and monitoring for asymptomatic ventricular dysfunction is recommended by some, there are at least two issues that clinicians should be aware of before screening asymptomatic patients. First, once identified, the significance of the subclinical ventricular dysfunction following cancer therapy is not known. Asymptomatic left ventricular systolic dysfunction in adults who have coronary artery disease has been associated with increased cardiovascular mortality, all-cause mortality, and progression to clinically overt CHF. It remains uncertain, however, whether these adverse outcomes can be extrapolated to young cancer survivors who have asymptomatic echocardiographic abnormalities. Second, it is not clear that long-term effective treatment is available for treatment-induced ventricular dysfunction. Although angiotensin-converting enzyme inhibitors have been shown to reduce the incidence of CHF in adult patients who have left ventricular dysfunction, their role in the treatment of subclinical cardiomyopathy among cancer survivors remains controversial [30,31].

Recognizing this, the COG recommends that patients treated with mediastinal RT or anthracyclines as children undergo echocardiography every 2 to 5 years depending on age of exposure and doses [7]. Radionuclide multiple-gated acquisition scanning is useful in individuals for whom good echocardiograms cannot be obtained. Patients who have evidence of valvular disease on echocardiography should be counseled regarding the need for prophylaxis for bacterial endocarditis.

Female survivors who have been treated during childhood with combined modality therapy or thoracic RT dose greater than 30 Gy or anthracyclines in doses exceeding 300 mg/m^2 should have echocardiographic evaluation in the third trimester of pregnancy, because symptomatic cardiac dysfunction may emerge during the substantial fluid load occurring at this time [7].

Coronary Artery Disease

Data are emerging that stress echocardiography may identify clinically important coronary artery disease in asymptomatic patients following mediastinal

RT. A recent prospective study reported the findings of 294 HL survivors previously treated with mediastinal RT who were screened with stress echocardiography and nuclear scintigraphy. All subjects were asymptomatic and had no known history of coronary artery disease [32]. The prevalence of severe, three-vessel, or left main coronary artery disease was 2.7%, with 7.5% of those treated with RT doses of 35 Gy or more having coronary stenosis greater than 50%. One notable finding in this study is that many survivors who had significant coronary artery disease did not have other cardiac risk factors, whereas most prior reports of cardiac mortality have not found this to be the case. The authors concluded that screening for coronary artery disease should be considered starting 5 years after completion of therapy for asymptomatic patients who have received mediastinal RT doses of 35 Gy or more [32].

Evaluation of Symptoms

Awareness of the increased risk for early-onset cardiovascular disease should illuminate the investigation of survivors who have chest pain, decline in exercise tolerance, or fatigue. Patients who have new onset of these symptoms should have echocardiographic evaluation of their valvular and ventricular function, and patients who have prior mediastinal RT should be referred to a cardiologist for consideration of stress testing to rule out significant coronary artery disease. Survivors in their 20s or 30s who were treated with cardiotoxic agents should not have heart disease discounted as a possible cause of these symptoms simply because of their young age. Similarly, there is a small increase in the risk for stroke or transient ischemic attacks among patients who received RT to the neck, and this diagnosis should be considered in survivors who experience neurologic symptoms, such as dizziness or visual changes, more than 5 years after this treatment.

DETECTION AND MANAGEMENT OF OTHER LATE EFFECTS

Thyroid Hormone Abnormalities

Hypothyroidism is the most common form of thyroid dysfunction occurring in HL survivors; within 20 years after completing radiation therapy, up to 50% of these patients may be affected with approximately half of cases occurring within 5 years. Radiation dose to the thyroid exceeding 20 to 30 Gy is the major risk factor [33]. Annual evaluation of thyroid stimulating hormone (TSH) should be started in the first year of follow-up to detect subclinical hypothyroidism among patients treated with neck RT. If TSH level becomes elevated then serum triiodothyronine (T3) and thyroxine (T4) should be evaluated to establish the degree of compensation. It is not necessary to initiate thyroid hormone replacement therapy at the first sign of TSH elevation. North American clinical practice guidelines recommend treatment in patients who have TSH levels greater than 10 μIU/mL or in patients who have TSH levels between 5 and 10 μIU/mL who also have a goiter or positive antithyroid peroxidase antibodies (or both), because these patients have the highest rates of progression to overt hypothyroidism [34].

Fertility and Ovarian Failure

Women treated with pelvic RT or alkylator-based chemotherapy regimens may experience irregular menses or premature menopause, and males may be oligo- or azoospermic. A full course (ie, six to eight cycles) of MOPP (mustine, vincristine, procarbazine, and prednisone), or dose-escalated BEACOPP (bleomycin, etoposide, doxorubicin, cyclophosphamide, vincristine, procarbazine, and prednisone) chemotherapy causes infertility in most survivors. ABVD alone seems to have little impact on fertility [35]. Male survivors treated at a young age may be unaware of their risks for infertility, and should be informed about this issue, with appropriate evaluation of sperm count and motility when indicated based on prior exposures and patients' informational needs. The use of hormonal therapy for females who have premature ovarian failure is unclear. In the setting of normal menopause, the USPSTF recommends against the routine use of combined estrogen and progestin for the prevention of chronic conditions [36]. The risk for breast cancer is significant for female HL survivors treated at a young age with mediastinal RT, and in view of evidence that estrogen replacement therapy may increase breast cancer risk in the general population it is generally not recommended for survivors who are already at increased risk. Menopausal vasomotor symptoms may be managed by nonhormonal therapy, or low-dose hormonal replacement may be undertaken after consultation with an appropriate specialist.

Infectious Complications

Excess mortality from infectious causes has been reported among HL survivors. In particular, patients who received RT to the spleen are generally considered to have functional asplenia, and less commonly a survivor may have had a surgical splenectomy. The Centers for Disease Control and Prevention recommends routine vaccination with pneumococcal and meningococcal polysaccharide vaccines in patients who have functional or anatomic asplenia, with revaccination after 5 years [37]. Some also recommend repeat *Haemophilus influenzae* b vaccination in these patients. With bacterial infections that might otherwise be easily manageable in an outpatient setting, asplenic patients can rapidly develop overwhelming sepsis. Those who develop fever greater than 101°F (38.3°C) should have blood cultures taken and be placed on broad-spectrum antibiotics, with careful monitoring [7].

Pulmonary Complications

Patients treated with bleomycin or mediastinal RT can have persistent abnormalities on pulmonary function tests (PFTs). Generally, these improve over time and are of no clinical consequence, although PFT results may not return to normal. One set of baseline tests 6 to 12 months after completion of therapy is worthwhile, although repeat PFTs in asymptomatic survivors is of limited value, because abnormal results generally do not lead to any useful intervention. In patients reporting shortness of breath, dyspnea on exertion, persistent cough, or recurrent pneumonia, however, it is appropriate to obtain PFTs and imaging studies. Reactive airway disease and asthma can be treated as they would in the general population, with referral to pulmonologists as needed for more complicated problems.

One unusual complication that can occur in patients previously treated with bleomycin is the emergence of significant pneumonitis shortly after exposure to supplemental oxygen, typically during surgical procedures. Although this is generally reported when oxygen is given within 12 months after bleomycin, significant pneumonitis has been reported up to 2 years later [38]. As a result of the recognized interaction between high-pressure oxygen and bleomycin and the potential severity of the resulting lung damage, some clinicians recommend that these survivors avoid scuba diving indefinitely, because it involves exposure to oxygen at high partial pressure [39], whereas others believe, based on clinical experience, that diving is safe 6 to 12 months after an uncomplicated course of bleomycin-containing chemotherapy [40].

Fatigue

Numerous studies have found that approximately one third of HL survivors experience persistent fatigue after treatment [41]. Fatigue seems to be more common following HL treatment than after treatment of leukemia or testicular cancer, and is associated with significant impairment of quality of life. A prospective study found that even before treatment patients who had early-stage HL had SF-36 vitality scores that were significantly below normal. The most significant predictor of posttreatment vitality score was the baseline score; complete response to treatment was not associated with normalization of energy levels [42].

Anemia and hypothyroidism should be ruled out in an HL survivor who is experiencing persistent fatigue after treatment. Fatigue has also been associated with cardiac complications in these survivors [43], and if not recently done, echocardiography should be undertaken to rule out ventricular or valvular dysfunction. Depression or insomnia should also be considered as a potential cause.

Once these modifiable medical causes have been ruled out, exercise is the most well-proven intervention to reduce fatigue in cancer survivors. Several trials have found that various forms of exercise can reduce cancer-related fatigue, with aerobic exercise likely providing the most benefit [41]. Some clinicians advise against weight lifting for patients treated with large cumulative doses of doxorubicin because of the increase in cardiovascular afterload that can occur with this activity. Support groups and psychosocial interventions may also be helpful in managing fatigue [41].

Several small trials have evaluated pharmacologic interventions to reduce cancer-related fatigue, generally in patients on treatment. Studies are often difficult to implement and interpret because of the higher-than-usual risk for creating a placebo effect when measuring fatigue. Methylphenidate has produced conflicting results compared with placebo in randomized trials. Modafinil is a stimulant used in the treatment of narcolepsy and other sleep disturbances. Two open-label studies of modafinil have found that the drug improves fatigue scores in patients who have breast cancer and brain tumors, and it is being evaluated in randomized controlled trials [44]. Data are emerging that proinflammatory cytokines, such as interleukin-6 and tumor necrosis factor-α, may play a role in fatigue in those on treatment and survivors [41]. These findings suggest that novel targeted agents may be developed to modulate the activity of these cytokines and reduce fatigue. Currently, however, pharmacotherapy for persistent fatigue in an HL survivor should probably be undertaken cautiously, after modifiable physiologic and psychologic causes have been ruled out.

SUMMARY

Advances in the treatment of HL have led to a significant improvement in long-term survival over the last 3 decades [1–3]. Reducing and managing the late effects of treatment are now major components of improving the overall outcome for these patients, particularly those diagnosed at young ages. Currently, recommendations for tailoring follow-up care to the specific risks for HL survivors are based on a knowledge of what these risks are and extrapolation from other clinical settings (Box 1). Recommendations for breast cancer screening, for example, are based on clear evidence of increased risk among certain HL survivors, and the knowledge that screen-detection of early breast cancer is feasible for other high-risk patients. It is increasingly recognized, however, that survivor-specific clinical trials are required to evaluate interventions that are now recommended largely based on common sense. As such trials develop, it should become possible to create programs of evidence-based follow-up care

---

Box 1: Routine tests recommended in the follow-up of Hodgkin lymphoma survivors

History and physical examination annually to include evaluation of cardiopulmonary function (eg, blood pressure), thyroid nodules

Complete blood count annually

TSH annually after neck RT, T3/T4 if TSH abnormal

Triglycerides, low-density lipoprotein and high-density lipoprotein cholesterol, fasting glucose every 2–3 years

Pneumococcal (re)vaccination every 5 years if treated with splenic RT or splenectomy; also meningococcal and *Haemophilus influenzae* vaccination

Cervical cancer screening according to established guidelines

Breast cancer screening annually starting 8–10 years after mediastinal RT if current age $\geq$25

Consider colorectal cancer screening starting at age 35–40 if $\geq$15 years after abdominal RT

Consider stress echocardiographic screening 5–10 years after mediastinal RT in adult survivors

Consider echocardiographic evaluation of ventricular/valvular function every 2–5 years after childhood exposure to anthracyclines or mediastinal RT.

for HL survivors. In view of the significant health problems experienced by some survivors, the resulting improvement in follow-up care will be an important step in improving the quality of life of patients cured of HL.

References

[1] van Spronsen DJ, Dijkema IM, Vrints LW, et al. Improved survival of Hodgkin's patients in south-east Netherlands since 1972. Eur J Cancer 1997;33(3):436–41.

[2] Kennedy BJ, Fremgen AM, Menck HR. The national cancer data base report on Hodgkin's disease for 1985-1989 and 1990-1994. Cancer 1998;83(5):1041–7.

[3] Hodgson DC, Zhang-Salomons J, Rothwell D, et al. Evolution of treatment for Hodgkin's disease: a population-based study of radiation therapy use and outcome. Clin Oncol (R Coll Radiol) 2003;15(5):255–63.

[4] Skinner R, Wallace WH, Levitt G. Therapy based long term follow up: practice statement. UK children's cancer study group. Available at: http://www.ukccsg.org.uk/public/followup/PracticeStatement/index.html; 2005. Accessed November 5, 2007.

[5] Scottish Intercollegiate Guidelines Network. Long term follow up of survivors of childhood cancer. Guideline no. 76. Available at: http://www.sign.ac.uk/pdf/sign76.pdf; 2004. Accessed November 5, 2007.

[6] NCCN Clinical Practice Guidelines in Oncology. Hodgkin disease/lymphoma. Available at: http://www.nccn.org/professionals/physician_gls/PDF/hodgkins.pdf; 2007. Accessed November 5, 2007.

[7] Children's Oncology Group. Long term follow-up guidelines. Available at: www.survivorshipguidelines.org; 2006. Accessed November 5, 2007.

[8] Deming RL, Constine LS, Elman AJ, et al. Follow-up of Hodgkin's disease. American College of Radiology. ACR appropriateness criteria. Radiology 2000;215(Suppl):1269–79.

[9] Aleman BM, van den Belt-Dusebout AW, Klokman WJ, et al. Long-term cause-specific mortality of patients treated for Hodgkin's disease. J Clin Oncol 2003;21(18):3431–9.

[10] Hodgson DC, Gilbert ES, Dores GM, et al. Long-term solid cancer risk among 5-year survivors of Hodgkin's lymphoma. J Clin Oncol 2007;25(12):1489–97.

[11] Hoppe RT. Hodgkin's disease: complications of therapy and excess mortality. Ann Oncol 1997;8:115–8.

[12] Travis LB, Hill DA, Dores GM, et al. Breast cancer following radiotherapy and chemotherapy among young women with Hodgkin disease. JAMA 2003;290(4):465–75.

[13] Swerdlow AJ, Schoemaker MJ, Allerton R, et al. Lung cancer after Hodgkin's disease: a nested case-control study of the relation to treatment. J Clin Oncol 2001;19(6):1610–8.

[14] Travis LB, Gilbert E. Lung cancer after Hodgkin lymphoma: the roles of chemotherapy, radiotherapy and tobacco use. Radiat Res 2005;163(6):695–6.

[15] Ralleigh G, Given-Wilson R. Breast cancer risk and possible screening strategies for young women following supradiaphragmatic irradiation for Hodgkin's disease. Clin Radiol 2004;59(8):647–50.

[16] Lee L, Pintilie M, Hodgson DC, et al. Screening mammography for young women treated with supradiaphragmatic radiation for Hodgkin's lymphoma. Annals of Oncology 2008;19:62–7.

[17] Diller L, Medeiros Nancarrow C, Shaffer K, et al. Breast cancer screening in women previously treated for Hodgkin's disease: a prospective cohort study. J Clin Oncol 2002;20(8):2085–91.

[18] Allen M, Ng A, Mauch P, et al. A decision and cost effectiveness analysis on tamoxifen as chemoprevention for breast cancer in young women treated with radiation therapy for Hodgkin's disease. Int J Radiat Oncol Biol Phys 2002;54(Suppl 1):11.

[19] Mauch P, Ng A, Aleman B, et al. Report from the Rockefeller foundation sponsored international workshop on reducing mortality and improving quality of life in long-term survivors of Hodgkin's disease. European J Haemotol 2005;75(Suppl 66):68–76.

[20] Henschke CI. CT screening for lung cancer is justified. Nat Clin Pract Oncol 2007;4(8): 440–1.

[21] Gleeson FV. Screening for lung cancer with spiral CT is not justified. Nat Clin Pract Oncol 2007;4(8):442–3.

[22] Das P, Ng AK, Earle CC, et al. Computed tomography screening for lung cancer in Hodgkin's lymphoma survivors: decision analysis and cost-effectiveness analysis. Ann Oncol 2006;17(5):785–93.

[23] Abrams DB, Raymond Niaura, Richard A, et al. The tobacco dependence treatment handbook: a guide to best practices. New York: Guilford Press; 2003.

[24] US Preventive Services Taskforce. Screening for colorectal cancer: recommendation and rationale. Ann Intern Med 2002;137(2):129–31.

[25] Colorectal cancer screening. Recommendation statement from the Canadian task force on preventive health care. CMAJ 2001;165(2):206–8.

[26] American Association of Clinical Endocrinologists and Associazione Medici Endocrinologi medical guidelines for clinical practice for the diagnosis and management of thyroid nodules. Endocr Pract 2006;12(1):63–102.

[27] Aleman BM, van den Belt-Dusebout AW, De Bruin ML, et al. Late cardiotoxicity after treatment for Hodgkin lymphoma. Blood 2007;109(5):1878–86.

[28] Hull MC, Morris CG, Pepine CJ, et al. Valvular dysfunction and carotid, subclavian, and coronary artery disease in survivors of Hodgkin lymphoma treated with radiation therapy. JAMA 2003;290(21):2831–7.

[29] Krischer JP, Epstein S, Cuthbertson DD, et al. Clinical cardiotoxicity following anthracycline treatment for childhood cancer: the pediatric oncology group experience. J Clin Oncol 1997;15(4):1544–52.

[30] Lipshultz SE, Lipsitz SR, Sallan SE, et al. Long-term enalapril therapy for left ventricular dysfunction in doxorubicin-treated survivors of childhood cancer. J Clin Oncol 2002;20(23): 4517–22.

[31] Silber JH, Cnaan A, Clark BJ, et al. Enalapril to prevent cardiac function decline in long-term survivors of pediatric cancer exposed to anthracyclines. J Clin Oncol 2004;22(5): 820–8.

[32] Heidenreich PA, Schnittger I, Strauss HW, et al. Screening for coronary artery disease after mediastinal irradiation for Hodgkin's disease. J Clin Oncol 2007;25(1):43–9.

[33] Constine LS, Donaldson SS, McDougall IR, et al. Thyroid dysfunction after radiotherapy in children with Hodgkin's disease. Cancer 1984;53(4):878–83.

[34] Gharib H, Tuttle RM, Baskin HJ, et al. Subclinical thyroid dysfunction: a joint statement on management from the American association of clinical endocrinologists, the American thyroid association, and the endocrine society. J Clin Endocrinol Metab 2005;90(1): 581–5 [discussion: 586–7].

[35] Hodgson DC, Pintilie M, Gitterman L, et al. Fertility among female Hodgkin lymphoma survivors attempting pregnancy following ABVD chemotherapy. Hematol Oncol 2007;25(1):11–5.

[36] Hormone therapy for the prevention of chronic conditions in postmenopausal women: recommendations from the U.S. Preventive Services task force. Ann Intern Med 2005;142(10):855–60.

[37] Bilukha OO, Rosenstein N. Prevention and control of meningococcal disease. Recommendations of the advisory committee on immunization practices (ACIP). MMWR Recomm Rep 2005;54(RR-7):1–21.

[38] Uzel I, Ozguroglu M, Uzel B, et al. Delayed onset bleomycin-induced pneumonitis. Urology 2005;66(1):195e.23–195e.25.

[39] Huls G, ten Bokkel Huinink D. Bleomycin and scuba diving: to dive or not to dive? Neth J Med 2003;61(2):50–3.

[40] de Wit R, Sleijfer S, Kaye SB, et al. Bleomycin and scuba diving: where is the harm? Lancet Oncol 2007;8(11):954–5.

[41] Ganz PA, Bower JE. Cancer related fatigue: a focus on breast cancer and Hodgkin's disease survivors. Acta Oncol 2007;46(4):474–9.

[42] Ganz PA, Moinpour CM, Pauler DK, et al. Health status and quality of life in patients with early-stage Hodgkin's disease treated on southwest oncology group study 9133. J Clin Oncol 2003;21(18):3512–9.

[43] Ng AK, Li S, Recklitis C, et al. A comparison between long-term survivors of Hodgkin's disease and their siblings on fatigue level and factors predicting for increased fatigue. Ann Oncol 2005;16(12):1949–55.

[44] Carroll JK, Kohli S, Mustian KM, et al. Pharmacologic treatment of cancer-related fatigue. Oncologist 2007;12(Suppl 1):43–51.

Testicular Cancer Patients: Considerations in Long-Term Follow-Up

Mary Gospodarowicz, MD, FRCPC, FRCR (Hon)[a,b,*]

[a]Department of Radiation Oncology, University of Toronto, Toronto, Ontario, Canada
[b]Cancer Program, Princess Margaret Hospital, 610 University Avenue, Toronto, Ontario M5G 2M9, Canada

O ver the past 30 years testicular tumors have become a paradigm for curable adult cancer. Numerous factors have contributed to this success. The introduction of tumor markers with beta human chorionic gonadotropin (β-HCG) and AFP contributed to more accurate diagnosis, staging, assessment of response, and monitoring of relapse. CT imaging led to improved staging of the retroperitoneum and chest and more accurate response assessment. In addition, the introduction of new treatment approaches with curative retroperitoneal lymph node dissection and highly effective cisplatin-based combination chemotherapy led to astounding cure rates in all stages of the disease [1].

These advances led to therapeutic approaches carefully adapted to the extent of disease [2–10]. Well-designed phase II and III clinical trials led to the development of surveillance protocols for stage I nonseminoma and seminoma [11,12]. Similarly, randomized phase III trials led to effective adjuvant strategies for stage II disease and optimal chemotherapeutic regimens for patients who had stage III disease.

Now, 30 years later, we have improved understanding of the pathogenesis of germ cell testis tumors and we are able to secure accurate pathologic diagnoses. Improved imaging methods depict accurately anatomic disease extent, and optimized use of surveillance, surgery, radiotherapy, and chemotherapy secures cure in 95% to 97% of all patients. Excellent survival rates have been documented in most European countries in the EUROCARE-4 study, with reduced variation in outcomes observed in the EUROCARE-3 study [13,14].

APPROACH TO OPTIMAL MANAGEMENT

In 2008, we owe each patient who has testis cancer a cure. To achieve a cure, efforts must be made to secure early diagnosis, arrive at precise diagnosis and staging, deliver high-quality expert treatment, minimize treatment exposure,

*Radiation Medicine Program, Princess Margaret Hospital, 610 University Avenue, Toronto, Ontario M5G 2M9, Canada. E-mail address: mary.gospodarowicz@rmp.uhn.on.ca

0889-8588/08/$ – see front matter
doi:10.1016/j.hoc.2008.01.003

and provide access to expert follow-up management. Even in the current era of extremely effective treatment, diagnostic delay results in inferior outcome. In a large population-based study in France, Huyghe and colleagues [15] demonstrated that diagnostic delay was associated with higher stage at presentation and had a significant adverse impact on survival in nonseminomas. No adverse outcome on survival was shown in seminoma. Because germ cell testis tumors are uncommon, there is limited opportunity to develop expertise in general oncology practice. Management in specialized cancer centers has been recommended, but this is not practical in all cases. Currently more than 70% of patients present with stage I disease and may be well managed following existing evidence-based practice guidelines, such as those developed in Europe, Canada, and in the United States by the National Comprehensive Cancer Network [4,6,10,16]. Less than 15% of patients present with stage III disease, however, and even today up to 50% of these patients will die of their disease. Expertise is needed in the management of these patients and in the management of patients who develop recurrent disease. Even large comprehensive cancer centers see only a limited number of these patients, and therefore maintenance of centers of excellence for the management of testis tumors, such as those established at Indiana University, Memorial Sloan-Kettering Cancer Center, and Royal Marsden Hospital in the United Kingdom, among others, are necessary.

It is important to optimize treatment approaches because increased therapeutic burden has been shown to carry additional toxicity and, in some cases, a higher late mortality. Sufficient knowledge and experience are available to minimize therapy without compromising cure. In stage I disease, the surveillance protocols introduced by Peckham and Horwich at Royal Marsden Hospital in late 1970s have matured with long-term outcome data from several different centers showing that delaying therapy until disease progression does not compromise cure [2–4,17–22]. Approximately 30% of stage I nonseminoma patients progress after orchiectomy. Those who have vascular invasion in the primary tumor carry a 50% risk for disease progression. Studies have shown that the use of adjuvant bleomycin, etopside, cisplatin chemotherapy virtually eliminates this risk but exposes 50% of patients unnecessarily to chemotherapy. In stage I seminoma, the risk for disease progression after orchiectomy is 15%.

The traditional approach to the management of stage I seminoma involved adjuvant radiation therapy (RT) with resulting 95% to 98% cure rate [3,4]. The acute toxicity of RT for stage I seminoma is low; treatment is well tolerated, and a dose of 25 Gy is sufficient to secure local control. Prospective studies have shown that RT can safely be limited to treating para-aortic lymph nodes and therefore many regard adjuvant retroperitoneal RT to be an extremely effective therapeutic intervention. Surveillance studies conducted over the past 20 years have shown that 85% of these patients are cured with orchiectomy alone, however, and therefore are exposed to RT unnecessarily. Currently, even the most ardent advocates of radiotherapy in stage I seminoma now offer surveillance to their patients.

FOLLOW-UP AFTER TREATMENT

Patients who achieve complete response following treatment, in general, are at low risk for relapse with the exception of patients on surveillance, in whom treatment is deferred by design to limit therapeutic exposure [23–26]. In addition, most patients who relapse manifest recurrent disease within 2 years following diagnosis. Late relapse has been reported and may occur as late as 30 years after the original diagnosis [27]. Such late relapse is extremely rare, however. In a large study, Oldenburg and colleagues from Norway found the cumulative 10-year incidence of late relapse to be 1.3% [25,26]. Late relapse may occur in both seminoma and nonseminoma. One of the relatively common scenarios is a late retroperitoneal relapse in nonseminoma treated without or with inadequate retroperitoneal lymph node dissection. Although the risk for late relapse is low, the management is not very successful with only 50% of patients who relapse with viable tumor surviving for 10 years [25].

In addition to late relapse, patients presenting with unilateral testicular tumor are at risk for developing a contralateral tumor, which may have the same or different histologic type. Contralateral testicular tumors have been diagnosed as late as 20 to 30 years following the diagnosis of the first tumor. The overall risk for contralateral testis tumor is low, however. In a large population-based study, Fossa and colleagues [28] showed the 15-year risk for contralateral testicular tumor to be 1.9%. Increasing age at diagnosis of first testicular cancer was associated with decreasing risk for metachronous contralateral testicular tumor. Second testis tumors are usually diagnosed at an early stage and are therefore highly curable. No formal screening for contralateral tumors is recommended, but raising awareness among testicular cancer survivors is advised [28].

LATE EFFECTS: OVERVIEW

Several textbooks and review articles provide detailed information on the late treatment effects in patients treated for testis tumors [29–41]. Increased risks for second cancers, including treatment-induced acute leukemia and solid second cancers, have been reported from many centers. Similarly, after the initial reports, several large studies documented the presence of cardiovascular morbidity following treatment and links to the metabolic syndrome. The most recent reports are highlighted below.

LATE EFFECTS: SECOND CANCERS

It has been known for decades that RT and chemotherapy lead to increased risks for second cancer. In the largest study to date, Travis and colleagues documented in a cohort of more than 40,000 patients who had testicular cancer 2285 second cancers when 1619 cancers were expected (observed/expected rate of 1.41) [40,42]. Increased cumulative risks for second cancers were observed in both seminoma and nonseminoma patients, and were more pronounced in patients who developed testis cancer at a younger age. Several other studies have now confirmed the increased second cancer risk in testicular tumors treated with RT [33,43–49]. These studies have led to renewed attention to minimizing treatment exposure with studies of surveillance, reduced dose and volume radiotherapy, and optimized chemotherapy regimens. Although treatment-induced leukemia is well documented following radiotherapy and chemotherapy in testicular tumors, fortunately its incidence is low [39,46]. Although extensive radiotherapy and cisplatin chemotherapy are associated with an increased risk for leukemia [39], most cases have been linked to treatment with high cumulative doses of topoisomerase II chemotherapy. Therapy-associated leukemias have been shown to be associated with etoposide-based chemotherapy. These leukemias develop 5 to 10 years after treatment and are characterized by chromosomal translocations involving bands 11q23 and 21q22 [46]. Approximately 0.5% of patients receiving cumulative doses less than 2 g of etoposide developed acute leukemia, whereas 2% of patients who received more than 2 g cumulative dose developed leukemia at 5 years posttreatment.

LATE EFFECTS: FERTILITY AND GONADAL TOXICITY

More than 50% of the patients who have testicular germ cell tumors have evidence of impaired spermatogenesis at diagnosis [34,35,50–53]. Cisplatin-based chemotherapy results in azoospermia immediately after therapy in most patients. This impairment is reversible in at least 50% of patients who receive standard-dose chemotherapy. Nevertheless, because at least half of patients do not recover fertility, sperm banking is recommended before treatment for all patients. Hypogonadism and androgen deficiency symptoms have been observed in 25% to 33% of patients [53]. Lower testosterone levels may play a part in the development of the metabolic syndrome observed in testis cancer survivors [37]. The introduction of nerve-sparing technique for retroperitoneal lymph node dissection virtually eliminated this form of morbidity [54].

LATE EFFECTS: NEUROTOXICITY, CARDIAC, METABOLIC SYNDROME, PULMONARY TOXICITY

The success of chemotherapy in curing germ cell testis cancers and the advances in symptom control with effective management of acute complications of nausea, vomiting, infections, and so on, have largely eliminated controversies in the management of active treatment for most patients. With growing numbers of long-term survivors of testis cancer, however, new knowledge of late-treatment effects is accumulating [29,30,50]. This knowledge is mandatory to guide the follow-up management of patients who have received chemotherapy. Cisplatin-based chemotherapy is the mainstay of successful treatment of germ cell testis tumors. Late effects of cisplatin chemotherapy include nephrotoxicity which, although frequently asymptomatic, is associated with up to 30% reduction in glomerular filtration rate [30,38,50,55,56]. Cisplatin-based peripheral neuropathy is characterized by paresthesias, tingling, and numbness and persists for several years in 20% to 40% of patients. Ototoxicity may include high-frequency hearing loss and tinnitus [57]. Up to 20% of patients report persistent symptoms. Cumulative dose of cisplatin seems to be correlated with the observed nephrotoxicity and ototoxicity.

In addition to the expected toxicity of chemotherapy and the well-known risk for second cancers following chemotherapy and radiotherapy, long-term follow-up of testicular cancer survivors has revealed increased risk for cardiovascular disease [29,36,41,58–60]. Raynaud phenomenon, hypertension, coronary artery disease with increase in angina pectoris, acute myocardial infarction, congestive heart failure, and peripheral vascular disease have been observed. In fact, the development of cardiovascular disease and increased risk for second cancers represent the most important long-term risks in patients cured of testicular cancer. The increased risk for cardiovascular disease has been related to direct endothelial damage and the metabolic syndrome. Follow-up studies of testicular cancer survivors revealed high incidence of increased serum cholesterol, dyslipidemia, obesity, and hypertension [61,62]. These risk factors together with insulin resistance are the main components of the metabolic syndrome [37,50,63–65]. The increased risk for metabolic syndrome has been shown in patients treated with chemotherapy and not in patients treated with surgery alone. Those treated with radiotherapy alone were at the same risk as patients treated with surgery alone. Serum testosterone level was inversely related to the presence of metabolic syndrome. It has been shown that smoking is associated with a higher risk for cardiovascular late effects.

Bleomycin administration has been associated with chronic lung injury that can result in lung fibrosis and, in rare instances, death. The toxicity of bleomycin is related to the cumulative dose, exposure to high oxygen concentrations, older age, and smoking [50,64].

LATE EFFECTS: QUALITY OF LIFE

Numerous studies document a relatively good quality of life in testicular cancer survivors [66]. Higher anxiety scores have been documented, however, with the youngest patients being most anxious [67,68]. No significant increase in depression scores was seen, other than in smokers [69]. Chronic fatigue may persist in some survivors. Sixteen percent of testicular cancer survivors suffer from fatigue as compared with a 10% fatigue rate in the general population [31,70].

SURVIVORSHIP CARE

The management of cancer survivors extends throughout the entire cancer journey and beyond [71]. The treatment of primary disease and then targeted follow-up leading to the early detection of any recurrence requires expertise and vigilance. The management of recurrence requires detailed information on previous presentations, prior treatments, and response to previous therapy. The management of the complications of cancer and its treatment can be intricate and lengthy. Those who require multiple therapeutic interventions may face cumulative treatment toxicities. In addition, currently, almost one in six cancer survivors overall will develop another cancer. Secondary prevention, screening, and early detection efforts are part of the management of all cancer survivors. The management of intercurrent disease requires familiarity with the previous cancer and details of its management [71]. Cancer survivors may suffer from residual anxiety and face numerous societal pressures related to difficulties with career, employment, and insurance. Follow-up strategies of testicular cancer survivors should focus on smoking cessation, management of the metabolic syndrome, and overall health maintenance [72].

Current guidelines for the management of testicular tumors focus on treatment recommendations [10,16]. Recognizing a small risk for late relapse, annual lifelong follow-up is suggested, but no evidence-based guidelines for the appropriate follow-up investigations are available. There is only one comprehensive review with recommendations for long-term medical care of testicular cancer survivors by Vaughn and colleagues [72]. It focuses on the primary care physician's evaluation and management of long-term survivors of testicular cancer treated with surgery and chemotherapy. It presents a useful guide to the care of testicular cancer survivors, recognizing that further information is required to optimally manage this complex group of patients.

Long-term sequelae of treatment are not uncommon in survivors of testicular tumors. Despite the recognition of the potential for multiple future health problems, the optimal long-term approach to care of these survivors and many other cancer survivor groups has not been defined. The 2005 report by the Institute of Medicine defined a desirable survivorship research agenda [73]. In addition, many recommendations were made for improved care of cancer survivors. An even more comprehensive set of recommendations was presented for survivorship research. Although the general recommendations presented in the Institute of Medicine report may be adapted to the management of testis cancer survivors, further research is urgently needed to optimize the long-term health maintenance strategies for survivors of testicular tumors (Box 1) [74,75].

There is evidence that patients and families faced with cancer are more receptive to health maintenance advice than the general population. This enhanced interest in health has been recognized as potential for dissemination of prevention and screening practices and deemed a "teachable moment" [76,77].

The low incidence of testicular cancer precludes any single institution's ability to have sufficiently broad experience to define standards of care for the follow-up of long-term survivors. International collaborative studies are required to gather sufficient data to generate information regarding standards of practice. The application of such standards will also be challenging. Testis cancer survivors represent a young, mobile population. It is unlikely that these patients will be available for single institution–based follow-up. It is more likely their long-term (20–30 or more years) care will be delivered by general practitioners with the guidance of Web-based information. These patients thus need to have direct access to their medical records and to top-level expertise.

Box 1: Recommendations from the Institute of Medicine and National Research Council Report

Raise awareness of the needs of survivors

Provide each patient with a Survivorship Care Plan

Develop evidence-based clinical practice guidelines

Develop quality of survivorship care measures

Provide support for demonstration programs to test models of coordinated, interdisciplinary survivorship care

Include consideration of survivorship in comprehensive cancer control plans

Provide educational opportunities to health care providers

Minimize adverse effects of cancer on employment

Provide access to adequate and affordable health insurance

Increase support of survivorship research

Data from Hewitt M, Greenfield S, Stovall M, editors. From cancer patient to cancer survivor: lost in transition. Institute of Medicine and National Research Council. Washington: National Academies Press; 2005.

Innovative strategies for survivorship interventions should include the use of modern information technologies, such as Web-based social networks, patient–survivor support groups, and other on-line communities [78–80]. The evolving role of e-health in reaching wide groups of health care consumers offers tremendous promise in enhancing the management of long-term cancer survivors [81–83]. Consumer informatics are changing the traditional relationship between providers of health care and patients [84,85]. Internet-based programs promise access to optimal expertise and should enable the overcoming of current geographic, economic, or social barriers [86–89].

References

[1] Bajorin DF. The graying of testis cancer patients: what have we learned? J Clin Oncol 2007;25(28):4341–3.

[2] Neill M, Warde P, Fleshner N. Management of low-stage testicular seminoma. Urol Clin North Am 2007;34(2):127–36 [abstract vii–viii].

[3] Albers P. Management of stage I testis cancer. Eur Urol 2007;51(1):34–43 [discussion: 43–4].

[4] Martin J, Chung P, Warde P. Treatment options, prognostic factors and selection of treatment in stage I seminoma. Onkologie 2006;29(12):592–8.

[5] Horwich A, Shipley J, Huddart R. Testicular germ-cell cancer. Lancet 2006;367(9512): 754–65.

[6] Albers P, Albrecht W, Algaba F, et al. Guidelines on testicular cancer. Eur Urol 2005;48(6): 885–94.

[7] Schmoll HJ, Souchon R, Krege S, et al. European consensus on diagnosis and treatment of germ cell cancer: a report of the European Germ Cell Cancer Consensus Group (EGCCCG). Ann Oncol 2004;15(9):1377–99.

[8] Jones RH, Vasey PA. Part II: testicular cancer—management of advanced disease. Lancet Oncol 2003;4(12):738–47.

[9] Jones RH, Vasey PA. Part I: testicular cancer—management of early disease. Lancet Oncol 2003;4(12):730–7.

[10] Krege S, Beyer J, Souchon R, et al. European Consensus Conference on Diagnosis and Treatment of Germ Cell Cancer: A Report of the Second Meeting of the European Germ Cell Cancer Consensus group (EGCCCG)-Part I. Eur Urol 2008;53(3):478–96.

[11] Milosevic MF, Gospodarowicz M, Warde P. Management of testicular seminoma. Semin Surg Oncol 1999;17(4):240–9.

[12] Raghavan D. Testicular cancer: maintaining the high cure rate. Oncology (Williston Park) 2003;17(2):218–28 [discussion: 228–9, 234–5], passim.

[13] Berrino F, De Angelis R, Sant M, et al. Survival for eight major cancers and all cancers combined for European adults diagnosed in 1995–99: results of the EUROCARE-4 study. Lancet Oncol 2007;8(9):773–83.

[14] Coleman MP, Gatta G, Verdecchia A, et al. EUROCARE-3 summary: cancer survival in Europe at the end of the 20th century. Ann Oncol 2003;14(Suppl 5):v128–49.

[15] Huyghe E, Muller A, Mieusset R, et al. Impact of diagnostic delay in testis cancer: results of a large population-based study. Eur Urol 2007;52(6):1710–6.

[16] http://www.nccn.org/professionals/physician_gls/PDF/testicular.pdf. page 1–31, Accessed March 13, 2008. (THE WHOLE DOCUMENT IS THE GUIDELINES)

[17] Peckham MJ, Hamilton CR, Horwich A, et al. Surveillance after orchiectomy for stage I seminoma of the testis. Br J Urol 1987;59(4):343–7.

[18] Peckham MJ, Barrett A, Horwick A, et al. Orchiectomy alone for Stage I testicular non-seminoma. A progress report on the Royal Marsden Hospital study. Br J Urol 1983;55(6):754–9.

[19] Chung P, Warde P. Surveillance in stage I testicular seminoma. Urol Oncol 2006;24(1):75–9.

[20] Warde P, Specht L, Horwich A, et al. Prognostic factors for relapse in stage I seminoma managed by surveillance: a pooled analysis. J Clin Oncol 2002;20(22):4448–52.

[21] Bayley A, Warde P, Milosevic M, et al. Surveillance for stage I testicular seminoma. a review. Urol Oncol 2001;6(4):139–43.

[22] Sturgeon JF, Jewett MA, Alison RE, et al. Surveillance after orchidectomy for patients with clinical stage I nonseminomatous testis tumors. J Clin Oncol 1992;10(4):564–8.

[23] Carver BS, Motzer RJ, Kondagunta GV, et al. Late relapse of testicular germ cell tumors. Urol Oncol 2005;23(6):441–5.

[24] Ehrlich Y, Baniel J. Late relapse of testis cancer. Urol Clin North Am 2007;34(2):253–8 [abstract x–xi].

[25] Oldenburg JM, Martin JM, Fossa SD. Late recurrences of germ cell malignancies: a population-based experience over three decades. Br J Cancer 2006;94(6):820–7.

[26] Oldenburg J, Martin JM, Fossa SD. Late relapses of germ cell malignancies: incidence, management, and prognosis. J Clin Oncol 2006;24(35):5503–11.

[27] Pavic M, Meeus P, Treilleux I, et al. Malignant teratoma 32 years after treatment of germ cell tumor confined to testis. Urology 2006;67(4):846, e11-3.

[28] Fossa SD, Chen J, Schonfeld SJ, et al. Risk of contralateral testicular cancer: a population-based study of 29,515 U.S. men. J Natl Cancer Inst 2005;97(14):1056–66.

[29] Abouassaly R, Klein EA, Raghavan D. Complications of surgery and chemotherapy for testicular cancer. Urol Oncol 2005;23(6):447–55.

[30] Boyer M, Raghavan D. Toxicity of treatment of germ cell tumors. Semin Oncol 1992;19(2):128–42.

[31] Fossa SD, Dahl AA, Loge JH. Fatigue, anxiety, and depression in long-term survivors of testicular cancer. J Clin Oncol 2003;21(7):1249–54.

[32] Fossa SD, Gilbert E, Dores GM, et al. Noncancer causes of death in survivors of testicular cancer. J Natl Cancer Inst 2007;99(7):533–44.

[33] Fossa SD, Langmark F, Aass N, et al. Second non-germ cell malignancies after radiotherapy of testicular cancer with or without chemotherapy. Br J Cancer 1990;61(4):639–43.

[34] Huddart RA, Norman A, Moynihan C, et al. Fertility, gonadal and sexual function in survivors of testicular cancer. Br J Cancer 2005;93(2):200–7.

[35] Huyghe E, Matsuda T, Daudin M, et al. Fertility after testicular cancer treatments: results of a large multicenter study. Cancer 2004;100(4):732–7.

[36] Kollmannsberger C, Kuzcyk M, Mayer F, et al. Late toxicity following curative treatment of testicular cancer. Semin Surg Oncol 1999;17(4):275–81.

[37] Nuver J, Smit AJ, Wolffenbuttel BH, et al. The metabolic syndrome and disturbances in hormone levels in long-term survivors of disseminated testicular cancer. J Clin Oncol 2005;23(16):3718–25.

[38] Strumberg D, Brugge S, Korn MW, et al. Evaluation of long-term toxicity in patients after cisplatin-based chemotherapy for non-seminomatous testicular cancer. Ann Oncol 2002;13(2):229–36.

[39] Travis LB, Andersson M, Gospodarowicz M, et al. Treatment-associated leukemia following testicular cancer. J Natl Cancer Inst 2000;92(14):1165–71.

[40] Travis LB, Fossa S, Schonfeld S, et al. Second cancers among 40,576 testicular cancer patients: focus on long-term survivors. J Natl Cancer Inst 2005;97(18):1354–65.

[41] van den Belt-Dusebout AW, de Wit R, Gietema JA, et al. Treatment-specific risks of second malignancies and cardiovascular disease in 5-year survivors of testicular cancer. J Clin Oncol 2007;25(28):4370–8.

[42] Travis LB, Curtis RE, Storm H, et al. Risk of second malignant neoplasms among long-term survivors of testicular cancer. J Natl Cancer Inst 1997;89(19):1429–39.

[43] Wierecky J, Kollmannsberger C, Boehlke I, et al. Secondary leukemia after first-line high-dose chemotherapy for patients with advanced germ cell cancer. J Cancer Res Clin Oncol 2005;131(4):255–60.

[44] Wanderas EH, Fossa SD, Tretli S. Risk of subsequent non-germ cell cancer after treatment of germ cell cancer in 2006 Norwegian male patients. Eur J Cancer 1997;33(2):253–62.

[45] van Leeuwen FE, Stiggelbout AM, van der Belt-Dusebout AW, et al. Second cancer risk following testicular cancer: a follow-up study of 1,909 patients. J Clin Oncol 1993;11(3):415–24.

[46] van Leeuwen FE. Risk of acute myelogenous leukaemia and myelodysplasia following cancer treatment. Baillieres Clin Haematol 1996;9(1):57–85.

[47] Richiardi L, Scelo G, Boffetta P, et al. Second malignancies among survivors of germ-cell testicular cancer: a pooled analysis between 13 cancer registries. Int J Cancer 2007;120(3):623–31.

[48] Kollmannsberger C, Hartmann JT, Kanz L, et al. Therapy-related malignancies following treatment of germ cell cancer. Int J Cancer 1999;83(6):860–3.

[49] Dong C, Hemminki K. Second primary neoplasms in 633,964 cancer patients in Sweden, 1958–1996. Int J Cancer 2001;93(2):155–61.

[50] Efstathiou E, Logothetis CJ. Review of late complications of treatment and late relapse in testicular cancer. J Natl Compr Canc Netw 2006;4(10):1059–70.

[51] Hartmann JT, Albrecht C, Schmoll HJ, et al. Long-term effects on sexual function and fertility after treatment of testicular cancer. Br J Cancer 1999;80(5–6):801–7.

[52] Jacobsen KD, Fossa SD, Bjoro TP, et al. Gonadal function and fertility in patients with bilateral testicular germ cell malignancy. Eur Urol 2002;42(3):229–38, discussion 237–8.

[53] Lackner JE, Mark I, Schatzl G, et al. Hypogonadism and androgen deficiency symptoms in testicular cancer survivors. Urology 2007;69(4):754–8.

[54] Fossa SD. Long-term sequelae after cancer therapy—survivorship after treatment for testicular cancer. Acta Oncol 2004;43(2):134–41.

[55] Hartmann JT, Kollmannsberger C, Kanz L, et al. Platinum organ toxicity and possible prevention in patients with testicular cancer. Int J Cancer 1999;83(6):866–9.

[56] Oh JH, Baum DD, Pham S, et al. Long-term complications of platinum-based chemotherapy in testicular cancer survivors. Med Oncol 2007;24(2):175–81.

[57] Bokemeyer C, Berger CC, Hartmann JT, et al. Analysis of risk factors for cisplatin-induced ototoxicity in patients with testicular cancer. Br J Cancer 1998;77(8):1355–62.

[58] Kohli S, Kohli M. Acute chemotherapy-induced cardiovascular changes in patients with testicular cancer: are there implications for blood pressure management in patients receiving chemotherapy? J Clin Oncol 2006;24(15):2399 [author reply 2399–400].

[59] Nuver J, Smit AJ, van der Meer J, et al. Acute chemotherapy-induced cardiovascular changes in patients with testicular cancer. J Clin Oncol 2005;23(36):9130–7.

[60] van den Belt-Dusebout AW, Nuver J, de Wit R, et al. Long-term risk of cardiovascular disease in 5-year survivors of testicular cancer. J Clin Oncol 2006;24(3):467–75.

[61] Sagstuen H, Aass N, Fossa SD, et al. Blood pressure and body mass index in long-term survivors of testicular cancer. J Clin Oncol 2005;23(22):4980–90.

[62] Raghavan D, Cox K, Childs A, et al. Hypercholesterolemia after chemotherapy for testis cancer. J Clin Oncol 1992;10(9):1386–9.

[63] Haugnes HS, Aass N, Fossa SD, et al. Components of the metabolic syndrome in long-term survivors of testicular cancer. Ann Oncol 2007;18(2):241–8.

[64] Kaufman MR, Chang SS. Short- and long-term complications of therapy for testicular cancer. Urol Clin North Am 2007;34(2):259–68 [abstract xi].

[65] de Haas EC, Sleijfer DT, Gietema JA. Follow-up of successfully treated testicular cancer patients: consequences of the metabolic syndrome. Ann Oncol 2007;18(2): 211–2.

[66] Mykletun A, Dahl AA, Haaland CF, et al. Side effects and cancer-related stress determine quality of life in long-term survivors of testicular cancer. J Clin Oncol 2005;23(13):3061–8.

[67] Dahl AA, Mykletun A, Fossa SD. Quality of life in survivors of testicular cancer. Urol Oncol 2005;23(3):193–200.

[68] Dahl AA, Haaland CF, Mykletun A, et al. Study of anxiety disorder and depression in long-term survivors of testicular cancer. J Clin Oncol 2005;23(10):2389–95.

[69] Shinn EH, Basen-Engquist K, Thornton B, et al. Health behaviors and depressive symptoms in testicular cancer survivors. Urology 2007;69(4):748–53.

[70] Joly F, Heron JF, Kalusinski L, et al. Quality of life in long-term survivors of testicular cancer: a population-based case-control study. J Clin Oncol 2002;20(1):73–80.

[71] Gospodarowicz M, O'Sullivan B. Patient management scenario: a framework for clinical decision and prognosis. Semin Surg Oncol 2003;21(1):8–12.

[72] Vaughn DJ, Gignac GA, Meadows AT. Long-term medical care of testicular cancer survivors. Ann Intern Med 2002;136(6):463–70.

[73] Hewitt M, Greenfield S, Stovall M, editors. From cancer patient to cancer survivor: lost in transition. Institute of Medicine and National Research Council. Washington: National Academies Press; 2005.

[74] Aziz NM. Cancer survivorship research: state of knowledge, challenges and opportunities. Acta Oncol 2007;46(4):417–32.

[75] Aziz NM, Rowland JH. Trends and advances in cancer survivorship research: challenge and opportunity. Semin Radiat Oncol 2003;13(3):248–66.

[76] Demark-Wahnefried W, et al. Riding the crest of the teachable moment: promoting long-term health after the diagnosis of cancer. J Clin Oncol 2005;23(24):5814–30.

[77] Ganz PA. A teachable moment for oncologists: cancer survivors, 10 million strong and growing!. J Clin Oncol 2005;23(24):5458–60.

[78] Doolittle GC, Spaulding A. Online cancer services: types of services offered and associated health outcomes. J Med Internet Res 2005;7(3):e35–6.

[79] Etter JF. A list of the most popular smoking cessation web sites and a comparison of their quality. Nicotine Tob Res 2006;8(Suppl 1):S27–34.

[80] Weiss JB, Campion TR Jr. Blogs, wikis, and discussion forums: attributes and implications for clinical information systems. Medinfo 2007;12(Pt 1):157–61.

[81] Oh H, Rizo C, Enkin M, et al. What is eHealth (3): a systematic review of published definitions. J Med Internet Res 2005;7(1):e1.

[82] Stjernsward S, Ostman M. Depression, e-health and family support. What the Internet offers the relatives of depressed persons. Nord J Psychiatry 2007;61(1):12–8.

[83] Jadad AR. A view from the Internet age: let's build a health system that meets the needs of the next generation. CMAJ 2004;171(12):1457–8.

[84] Anderson JG, Rainey MR, Eysenbach G. The impact of CyberHealthcare on the physician-patient relationship. J Med Syst 2003;27(1):67–84.

[85] Eysenbach G, Jadad AR. Evidence-based patient choice and consumer health informatics in the Internet age. J Med Internet Res 2001;3(2):E19.

[86] Boulos MN, Maramba I, Wheeler S. Wikis, blogs and podcasts: a new generation of Web-based tools for virtual collaborative clinical practice and education. BMC Med Educ 2006;6:41.

[87] Winefield HR. Support provision and emotional work in an Internet support group for cancer patients. Patient Educ Couns 2006;62(2):193–7.

[88] Eysenbach G, Powell J, Englesakis M, et al. Health related virtual communities and electronic support groups: systematic review of the effects of online peer to peer interactions. Bmj 2004;328(7449):1166.

[89] Eysenbach G. From intermediation to disintermediation and apomediation: new models for consumers to access and assess the credibility of health information in the age of Web2.0. Medinfo 2007;12(Pt 1):162–6.

The Genetics of Cancer Survivorship

James M. Allan, DPhil

Northern Institute for Cancer Research, Paul O'Gorman Building, Medical School, Framlington Place, Newcastle University, Newcastle upon Tyne NE2 4HH, UK

The probability of surviving cancer is determined by numerous interacting genotypic, phenotypic, and treatment-related characteristics. Research efforts have traditionally focused on phenotypic characteristics, such as age, comorbidities, and stage of disease [1], and treatment-related characteristics, such as dosing regimen [2]. More recently it has become apparent that genetics, including constitutional (host-related hereditary) and acquired somatic (disease-specific) genetics, can also have a major impact on cancer outcome and survivorship. Importantly, constitutional and somatic genetics can affect cancer outcome at several points during the natural history of disease, including cancer progression, induction death, chemoresistant disease, relapsing disease, and the risk for developing comorbidities and other long-term adverse effects.

ACQUIRED SOMATIC GENETICS AND CANCER SURVIVORSHIP

The development of novel therapies for the treatment of malignancy has focused on taking advantage of features unique to disease; therapies are targeted specifically against acquired phenotypic or genotypic characteristics unique to the neoplastic clone. For example, fusion of the *breakpoint cluster region* (*BCR*) gene on chromosome 22 and the *abelson* (*ABL*) tyrosine kinase gene on chromosome 9 gives rise to the Philadelphia chromosome harboring the *BCR-ABL* fusion gene, with constitutively active tyrosine kinase activity of the expressed fusion protein [3]. The Philadelphia translocation is characteristic of chronic myeloid leukemia (CML), and is also reported in acute lymphoblastic and acute myeloid leukemia (AML) [4]. Targeted therapy using tyrosine kinase inhibitors, such as imatinib mesylate, are effective against leukemias expressing the *BCR-ABL* fusion gene and have significantly improved patient outcome [5,6]. Similarly, the t(15;17) translocation in AML fuses the *retinoic acid receptor alpha* (*RARalpha*) gene on chromosome 15 to the *promyelocytic leukemia* (*PML*) gene on chromosome 17, giving rise to acute promyelocytic leukemia (APL), which is responsive to differentiation therapy using all-trans retinoic

JMA gratefully acknowledges the support of Leukaemia Research, Yorkshire Cancer Research, Cancer Research UK, and the Candlelighters' Trust.

E-mail address: james.allan@newcastle.ac.uk

acid [7]. As a consequence of targeted therapy, APL has emerged as the most curable form of AML; up to 80% of adult patients can be cured with treatment that includes retinoic acid and anthracyclines [8]. The efficacy of retinoic acid is a direct consequence of an effect on leukemic blasts, which are selectively driven toward terminal differentiation by virtue of the expressed *APL-RARalpha* fusion gene [8]. Treatment of *BCR-ABL*–positive leukemias with tyrosine kinase inhibitors and t(15;17)-positive APL with retinoic acid are paradigms of targeted therapy in hematologic disease in which the diagnosis of an overt cytogenetic alteration indicates treatment and determines outcome and survivorship.

Approximately 60% of AML cases are characterized by an overt karyotypic abnormality [9,10], and these remain a marker of patient prognosis [10,11]. In addition to t(15;17)-positive leukemia, myeloid disease characterized by inv16 or t(8;21) also has a generally favorable outcome, whereas AML characterized by monosomy of chromosomes 5 or 7, long-arm deletions of chromosome 5, 3q alterations, or a complex karyotype with five or more independent alterations generally have a poor outcome by comparison [10–13]. The remaining patients, including those who have a normal karyotype, have an intermediate outcome [10–13]. Like myeloid disease, good risk and poor risk cytogenetic subgroups can be identified in B-cell leukemias [14,15], and these can be used to direct therapy in adult patients and children [16,17]. Global gene expression analysis can be used to cluster myeloid leukemias by karyotype without any prior knowledge of abnormality [18–20], demonstrating that such abnormalities define the overt biology of the leukemic clone. Taken together, these data suggest that for many leukemias the presence of an overt karyotypic abnormality has a major effect on disease biology and ultimately on outcome and survivorship.

Despite considerable evidence demonstrating a role for overt karyotype in determining disease biology, even within these well-defined disease subgroups there remains considerable heterogeneity in disease outcome and overall survival. For example, AML with a normal karyotype, which represents approximately 40% of cases, is highly heterogeneous with respect to prognosis. In support of this, gene expression profiling of leukemic blast cells identified distinct subgroups with significantly different outcomes [19,20]. These and other data prompted an intensified search for subcytogenetic somatic alterations responsible for the clinical heterogeneity in AML, with considerable success. Several studies have shown that internal tandem duplications or point mutations in the *FLT3* gene, which encodes a tyrosine kinase, are common in AML and that these are independent prognostic markers in some disease subtypes [21–26]. Subcytogenetic alterations affecting other genes also add important prognostic information to a diagnosis of AML, including *WT1* [27], *CEBPA* [28], *KIT* [25,29], and *NPM1* [30,31].

The molecular genetics underlying the pathogenesis of AML is perhaps better understood than any other human cancer. As a consequence, the development of targeted therapies for disease subtypes defined at the subcytogenetic level (and the cytogenetic level) is now becoming a reality, including FLT3 tyrosine kinase inhibitors [32–34]. The development of targeted therapies for genetically characterized disease can result in dramatic improvements in long-term cancer survival, as illustrated by the examples of APL and CML. By extrapolation, we can predict that elucidating the somatic genetics underlying other hematologic diseases and also solid malignancies will lead to the development of other targeted therapies, improved patient outcome, and increasing numbers of cancer survivors. Given this, we can predict that acquired somatic genetics will become increasingly important as a determinant of cancer survivorship.

Like somatic genetics at presentation, alterations acquired at disease relapse can also affect outcome and have significant implications for survivorship. The potential impact of acquired somatic genetics on outcome is illustrated by the example of relapsing CML. Treatment of Philadelphia-positive CML in chronic phase with imatinib mesylate induces a complete cytogenetic response in more than 80% of cases, but the *BCR-ABL* fusion is still detectable using molecular techniques in most of these cases [35]. Unfortunately, as a consequence of acquired point mutations in the kinase domain of BCR-ABL, many patients who have CML relapse with disease that is resistant to imatinib mesylate [36]. This phenomenon is typified by the example of the T315I mutation. This and other kinase domain mutations give rise to a chimeric protein with altered conformation [37], such that interaction with imatinib mesylate at the molecular level is physically impaired. The development of clinical resistance has stimulated the development of second-generation tyrosine kinase inhibitors with efficacy in patients who have imatinib mesylate–resistant disease [38], although treatment of T315I-mutated chronic myeloid leukemia remains highly problematic [39].

As a parallel to targeted therapy that takes advantage of somatically acquired disease-specific alterations, research efforts have also focused on the development of therapeutic strategies individualized to the patient. This approach recognizes that response to cancer therapy and outcome may be independent of disease (as well as being disease dependent), and that constitutional genetics common to neoplastic and nonneoplastic cells can significantly affect survival.

CONSTITUTIONAL GENETICS AND CANCER SURVIVORSHIP

The human genome is highly polymorphic and includes an estimated 10 million single nucleotide polymorphisms [40] in addition to numerous structural alterations, such as deletions, duplications, and large-scale copy number variants [41]. Attempts to elucidate the contribution of constitutional genetic variation to survival following a diagnosis of cancer have traditionally focused on genes in cellular pathways that modify chemotherapy drug metabolism or detoxification. For example, reactive metabolites of several chemotherapeutic alkylating agents are subject to cellular phase II detoxification by way of conjugation to glutathione, mediated by cytosolic glutathione S-transferases, including glutathione S-transferase P1 (GSTP1) [42]. GSTP1 is encoded by a single locus on chromosome 11 (*GSTP1*) that displays allelic variation in humans. A common single nucleotide polymorphism at codon 105 in exon 5 results in an isoleucine to valine substitution. Codon 105 forms part of the active site for binding of reactive electrophiles, and the valine substitution encodes a protein with reduced conjugation activity and lower thermal stability, relative to the isoleucine-containing variant at codon 105 [42,43]. There is convincing evidence that the codon 105 variant affects outcome following treatment with chemotherapeutic alkylating agents, in which therapy includes agents conjugated by GSTP1, including colon cancer [44,45], multiple myeloma [46], gastric cancer [47], Hodgkin lymphoma [48], and breast cancer [49]. In addition to genetic variation in pathways that affect drug metabolism, outcome studies have also focused on candidate genes in pathways that affect drug absorption, renal excretion, and cellular response to genotoxic damage, such as DNA repair [50]. As a consequence of recent developments in single nucleotide polymorphism genotyping technology, however, there is an ongoing shift of emphasis away from candidate gene- and pathway-based studies toward genome-wide studies with the potential to type millions of variants simultaneously. This approach is likely to identify numerous potentially interacting constitutional genetic variants with an important role in determining cancer survivorship.

In addition to investigating the constitutional genotype, use of this technology to interrogate the somatic genome has also identified allelic deletion, uniparental disomy (allelic deletion with reconstitution to the diploid state by way of recombination and duplication of the remaining allele), microdeletions, and gene amplification as common events in cancer. Many of these alterations, particularly uniparental disomy and allelic deletion, frequently affect large regions of the genome [51–54]. These events result in a polymorphism profile in cancer cells that is markedly different from the constitutional genotype, including heterozygous polymorphisms being rendered homozygous.

GENETICS, NATURAL HISTORY OF DISEASE, AND SURVIVORSHIP

Although the effect of somatically acquired genetics on cancer survival is disease-specific, understanding the influence of constitutional genetics of cancer survivorship is intrinsically more difficult because any effect could potentially be both disease dependent and disease independent. Moreover, constitutional and somatic genetics can affect outcome at multiple points during the natural history of disease, including disease progression, induction death, resistant disease, remission failure, disease relapse, and risk for life-threatening comorbidities and other long-term effects (Fig. 1). Ultimately, each of these features can significantly affect cancer survivorship. This principle can be illustrated using examples taken from the study of hematologic malignancy.

Chronic lymphocytic leukemia (CLL) can present as a relatively indolent disease, for which treatment is not always indicated at diagnosis but may be recommended with the onset of progressive disease, sometimes several years after diagnosis. Somatic mutation in the variable region of the immunoglobulin heavy chain locus (IgV_H) is closely correlated with disease progression [55];

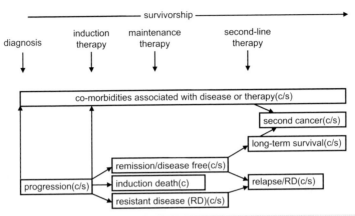

Fig. 1. Constitutional and somatic genetics, natural history of disease, and survivorship. This figure illustrates the basic natural history of disease and how constitutional (c) genetics and somatic genetics (s) impact on outcome and survivorship following a diagnosis of cancer. It should be noted that constitutional (c) refers to genetic variation common to neoplastic and non-neoplastic cells, whereas somatic (s) refers to genetic alterations acquired during the transformation process. Although it is likely that constitutional genetics plays a major role in defining risk for induction death, a direct role for somatic genetics cannot be excluded; RD, resistant disease.

patients who have a greater than 98% homology to constitutional sequence experience progressive disease requiring earlier treatment compared with patients who have CLL that presents with mutated IgV_H (less than 98% homology to constitutional sequence). As such, overall survival of patients who have unmutated CLL is considerably shorter (median is approximately 8 years for stage A patients) compared with those who have mutated CLL (median is greater than 20 years for stage A patients) [55]. Given the indolent nature of CLL it is perhaps not surprising that genetic markers affecting progression to an aggressive phenotype have such a major impact on overall survival and that overall survival in CLL is to a large extent independent of treatment. CLL serves as a paradigm for other indolent or low-grade hematologic diseases, such as non-Hodgkin lymphoma (NHL). Like CLL, treatment of low-grade NHL is often indicated at diagnosis, and there is no survival disadvantage if treatment is delayed until the onset of clinical progression [56]. In contrast to CLL and NHL, however, outcome following a diagnosis of many other malignancies is currently determined predominantly by host and disease response to therapy.

Although therapy can improve cancer survivorship, such an approach can also be associated with severe toxicity and induction death and can have a significant impact on cancer survivorship. Thiopurine prodrugs, such as 6-mercaptopurine and azathioprine, are used extensively to treat malignant disease, including myeloid and lymphoblastic leukemia. Clinical efficacy depends on activation to thioguanine nucleotides, such as 6-thioguanine, which promote cell death when incorporated into nucleic acids (reviewed by Coulthard and Hogarth [57]). Thioguanine nucleotides are subject to S-methylation and detoxification by thiopurine S-methyltransferase (TPMT) [57,58]. TPMT activity in humans displays considerable heterogeneity, with approximately 90% of humans having high activity, 10% having intermediate activity, and 0.3% having very low or null activity. This phenotypic heterogeneity is the result of a high degree of constitutional genetic variation in the *TPMT* gene [59]. Eight major *TPMT* alleles have been identified, with three of these (*TPMT2, TPMT3A,* and *TPMT3C*) accounting for approximately 90% of all intermediate-, low-, and null-activity cases. Individuals homozygous or compound heterozygous for *TPMT2, TPMT3A,* or *TPMT3C* are null for TPMT activity, whereas heterozygotes (with one wild-type allele) have intermediate TMPT activity [60]. TPMT activity is a critical determinant of patient response to thiopurine-based therapy. Treatment of low- or null-activity patients with standard-dose thiopurine therapy can lead to acute bone marrow toxicity and induction death attributable to neutropenia [61,62]. Constitutional *TPMT* genotype is thus a major risk determinant for induction death; routine genetic screening before administration of thiopurine chemotherapy and appropriate dose modification for low- and null-activity patients is indicated [63]. Similarly, induction death is a significant cause of treatment failure in patients treated with retinoic acid for APL, in which 10% to 15% of patients experience often fatal hemorrhage [64]. Although the underlying risk factors remain unidentified it is likely that constitutional genetic variation plays a major part.

Failure to achieve remission induction can also arise as a consequence of chemoresistant disease. There is considerable evidence to suggest that both constitutional and somatic genetics can determine disease sensitivity to induction therapy. For example, the t(8;21) translocation gives rise to myeloid leukemia that is relatively chemosensitive and is associated with a favorable outcome as a result [10]. Cell model systems have revealed that transcriptional activity of the AML1-ETO chimeric oncoprotein (generated as a consequence of the t(8;21) translocation) gives rise to down-regulation of cellular DNA repair activity, with concomitant up-regulation of the P53 proapoptotic pathway [65]. Taken together, these features are predicted to result in a leukemic clone that is sensitive to the killing effects of chemotherapy, and go some way toward explaining the relatively good response to induction therapy and favorable outcome of t(8;21)-positive AML [10]. Likewise, constitutionally determined DNA repair and apoptotic activity can also affect cellular response to therapy and outcome. For example, a common polymorphism (codon 751, lysine → glutamine) in xeroderma pigmentosum group D (XPD), a component of nucleotide excision DNA repair (NER), significantly predicted disease-free survival in elderly patients treated for AML, with a concomitant effect on overall survival [50]. The effect of the codon 751 variant on outcome was restricted to risk for relapse and was not associated with resistant disease, induction death, or remission (Table 1) [50]. The use of a chemotherapeutic nitrogen mustard (predicted to induce DNA damage repaired by NER) as maintenance therapy but not induction therapy in this series of AML patients might explain why the effect of this variant is restricted to disease-free survival. Park and colleagues [66]

Table 1
Association between the XPD codon 751 polymorphism (lysine→glutamine) and the outcome of patients after chemotherapy who have acute myeloid leukemia

XPD codon 751 status	All cases	Complete remission	Resistant disease	Induction death	Disease-free survival at 12 months	Overall survival at 12 months
All patients, N (%)	341 (100)	189 (55)	83 (24)	69 (20)	125 (37)	118 (35)
Lys/Lys, N (%)	134 (100)	75 (56)	29 (22)	30 (22)	59 (44)	51 (38)
Lys/Gln, N (%)	163 (100)	94 (58)	42 (26)	27 (17)	59 (36)	57 (35)
Gln/Gln, N (%)	44 (100)	20 (45)	12 (27)	12 (27)	7 (15)	10 (22)
P value		.8	.8	1.0	.04[a]	.07[a]

All P values are for trend.
Abbreviations: Gln, glutamine; Lys, lysine.
[a]Analysis adjusted for cytogenetic status, age, performance status, and white blood cell count.
Data from Allan JM, Smith AG, Wheatley K, et al. Genetic variation in XPD predicts treatment outcome and risk of acute myeloid leukemia following chemotherapy. Blood 2004;104:3875.

reported a similar association between the *XPD* codon 751 variant and overall survival in patients who had colorectal cancer, but in this study the association with outcome was related to initial tumor response to first-line therapy with platinum-based therapy, which also induces DNA damage recognized and repaired by NER [67]. In contrast, two subsequent studies reported a lack of association between the codon 751 variant and overall survival in pediatric and adult patients who had AML [68,69]. Induction and maintenance treatment protocols used in these studies did not include any agents known or predicted to induce DNA damage repaired by NER, however. These data highlight two important issues. First, any potential effect of genetics on survivorship must be considered in the context of other factors, including therapy, for example, but also host and disease characteristics. Second, genetics can impact on survivorship at multiple points during the natural history of disease, including initial disease response to therapy and also risk for relapse (see Fig. 1).

We must also consider the possibility that genetics, particularly constitutional genetics, influence long-term comorbidities that also have a significant impact on survivorship (see Fig. 1). For example, infections are a major feature in the clinical course of CLL and are a significant cause of death [70]. Along with immune dysfunction associated with disease, several alkylating agents that have been used to treat CLL also induce immune suppression [71], and it is plausible that genetic modifiers of drug metabolism and cellular response, including those discussed above, could have a major impact on patient susceptibility to opportunistic pathogens and risk for sepsis-related death. Moreover, there is substantial evidence that genetics can impact significantly on other long-term adverse events, including development of a potentially fatal therapy-induced malignancy. The codon 105 variant of GSTP1 has been associated with a significantly increased risk for developing chemotherapy-induced acute myeloid leukemia (t-AML) (Table 2) [72]. Predictably, risk was highest in

Table 2

Association between the glutathione S-transferase P1 codon 105 polymorphism (isoleucine→valine) and risk for therapy-induced acute myeloid leukemia

GSTP1 codon 105	de novo AML, N (%)	t-AML, N (%) (all cases)	Odds ratio (95% CI)	t-AML, N (%) (postchemotherapy)	Odds ratio (95% CI)	t-AML, N (%) (post GSTP1 substrates)	Odds ratio (95% CI)[a]
Iso/Iso	202 (49)	33 (37)	1 (–)	14 (27)	1 (–)	4 (19)	1 (–)
Iso/Val	151 (36)	40 (45)	1.87 (1.11–3.17)	28 (55)	2.87 (1.45–5.67)	12 (57)	4.43 (1.39–14.12)
Val/Val	61 (15)	16 (18)	1.67 (0.84–3.30)	9 (18)	2.17 (0.89–5.29)	5 (24)	4.16 (1.07–16.07)
Iso/Val + Val/Val	212 (51)	56 (63)	1.81 (1.11–2.94)	37 (73)	2.66 (1.39–5.09)	17 (81)	4.34 (1.43–13.20)

Abbreviations: AML, acute myeloid leukemia; CI, confidence interval; Iso, isoleucine; t-AML, therapy-induced acute myeloid leukemia; Val, valine.

[a]Odds ratios and 95% confidence intervals were calculated using unconditional logistic regression and using de novo AML cases as the reference.

Data from Allan JM, Wild CP, Rollinson S, et al. Polymorphism in glutathione S-transferase P1 is associated with susceptibility to chemotherapy-induced leukemia. Proc Natl Acad Sci U S A 2001;98:11596.

patients previously treated with chemotherapy agents that are substrates for glutathione conjugation by GSTP1 (see Table 2) [72]. It is biologically plausible that the GSTP1 codon 105 variant has a direct impact on susceptibility to mutation and transformation in non-target bone marrow progenitor cells, conferring susceptibility to t-AML. We must also consider the possibility, however, that the population at risk for developing a therapy-induced cancer is genetically biased for this variant because of its role as a prognostic marker after treatment of primary cancer, including colon cancer [44,45], multiple myeloma [46], gastric cancer [47], Hodgkin lymphoma [48], and breast cancer [49]. Genetic susceptibility to iatrogenic malignancies is also complicated by other factors, and these have been reviewed elsewhere [73].

SUMMARY

Host and disease phenotype at presentation are critical determinants of outcome and survival following a diagnosis of cancer. Given that phenotype is determined to a large extend by genotype it is perhaps not surprising that genetics should also play an important role in defining outcome and survivorship. A better understanding of constitutional and somatic genetics will allow for therapeutic regimens to be individualized to the patient and for the development of therapies targeted against specific disease types. Advances in our understanding of genetics, in conjunction with the development of more sophisticated therapies and treatment regimens, can only become more important as a pivotal determinant of survivorship.

References
[1] Lossos IS, Morgensztern D. Prognostic biomarkers in diffuse large B-cell lymphoma. J Clin Oncol 2006;24(6):995–1007.
[2] Kolitz JE. Current therapeutic strategies for acute myeloid leukaemia. Br J Haematol 2006;134(6):555–72.
[3] Mauro MJ, Druker BJ. Chronic myelogenous leukemia. Curr Opin Oncol 2001;13(1):3–7.
[4] Cilloni D, Guerrasio A, Giugliano E, et al. From genes to therapy: the case of Philadelphia chromosome-positive leukemias. Ann N Y Acad Sci 2002;963:306–12.
[5] Druker BJ, Talpaz M, Resta DJ, et al. Efficacy and safety of a specific inhibitor of the BCR-ABL tyrosine kinase in chronic myeloid leukemia. N Engl J Med 2001;344(14):1031–7.
[6] Mauro MJ, Druker BJ. STI571: targeting BCR-ABL as therapy for CML. Oncologist 2001;6(3):233–8.
[7] Mistry AR, Pedersen EW, Solomon E, et al. The molecular pathogenesis of acute promyelocytic leukaemia: implications for the clinical management of the disease. Blood Rev 2003;17(2):71–97.
[8] Tallman MS. Acute promyelocytic leukemia as a paradigm for targeted therapy. Semin Hematol 2004;41(2 Suppl 4):27–32.
[9] Bacher U, Kern W, Schnittger S, et al. Population-based age-specific incidences of cytogenetic subgroups of acute myeloid leukemia. Haematologica 2005;90(11):1502–10.
[10] Grimwade D, Walker H, Oliver F, et al. The importance of diagnostic cytogenetics on outcome in AML: analysis of 1,612 patients entered into the MRC AML 10 trial. The Medical Research Council Adult and Children's Leukaemia Working Parties. Blood 1998;92(7):2322–33.
[11] Grimwade D, Moorman A, Hills R, et al. Impact of karyotype on treatment outcome in acute myeloid leukemia. Ann Hematol 2004;83(Suppl 1):S45–8.

[12] Grimwade D. The clinical significance of cytogenetic abnormalities in acute myeloid leukae-mia. Best Pract Res Clin Haematol 2001;14(3):497–529.

[13] Grimwade D, Walker H, Harrison G, et al. The predictive value of hierarchical cytogenetic classification in older adults with acute myeloid leukemia (AML): analysis of 1065 patients entered into the United Kingdom Medical Research Council AML11 trial. Blood 2001;98(5):1312–20.

[14] Moorman AV, Harrison CJ, Buck GA, et al. Karyotype is an independent prognostic factor in adult acute lymphoblastic leukemia (ALL): analysis of cytogenetic data from patients treated on the Medical Research Council (MRC) UKALLXII/Eastern Cooperative Oncology Group (ECOG) 2993 trial. Blood 2007;109(8):3189–97.

[15] Moorman AV, Richards SM, Robinson HM, et al. Prognosis of children with acute lympho-blastic leukemia (ALL) and intrachromosomal amplification of chromosome 21 (iAMP21). Blood 2007;109(6):2327–30.

[16] Pui CH, Evans WE. Treatment of acute lymphoblastic leukemia. N Engl J Med 2006;354(2): 166–78.

[17] Piccaluga PP, Paolini S, Martinelli G. Tyrosine kinase inhibitors for the treatment of Philadel-phia chromosome-positive adult acute lymphoblastic leukemia. Cancer 2007;110(6): 1178–86.

[18] Heuser M, Wingen LU, Steinemann D, et al. Gene-expression profiles and their association with drug resistance in adult acute myeloid leukemia. Haematologica 2005;90(11): 1484–92.

[19] Valk PJ, Verhaak RG, Beijen MA, et al. Prognostically useful gene-expression profiles in acute myeloid leukemia. N Engl J Med 2004;350(16):1617–28.

[20] Bullinger L, Dohner K, Bair E, et al. Use of gene-expression profiling to identify prognostic subclasses in adult acute myeloid leukemia. N Engl J Med 2004;350(16):1605–16.

[21] Kottaridis PD, Gale RE, Linch DC. Prognostic implications of the presence of FLT3 mutations in patients with acute myeloid leukemia. Leuk Lymphoma 2003;44(6):905–13.

[22] Kottaridis PD, Gale RE, Frew ME, et al. The presence of a FLT3 internal tandem duplication in patients with acute myeloid leukemia (AML) adds important prognostic information to cyto-genetic risk group and response to the first cycle of chemotherapy: analysis of 854 patients from the United Kingdom Medical Research Council AML 10 and 12 trials. Blood 2001;98(6):1752–9.

[23] Schnittger S, Schoch C, Dugas M, et al. Analysis of FLT3 length mutations in 1003 patients with acute myeloid leukemia: correlation to cytogenetics, FAB subtype, and prognosis in the AMLCG study and usefulness as a marker for the detection of minimal residual disease. Blood 2002;100(1):59–66.

[24] Boissel N, Cayuela JM, Preudhomme C, et al. Prognostic significance of FLT3 internal tandem repeat in patients with de novo acute myeloid leukemia treated with reinforced courses of chemotherapy. Leukemia 2002;16(9):1699–704.

[25] Boissel N, Leroy H, Brethon B, et al. Incidence and prognostic impact of c-Kit, FLT3, and Ras gene mutations in core binding factor acute myeloid leukemia (CBF-AML). Leukemia 2006;20(6):965–70.

[26] Stirewalt DL, Kopecky KJ, Meshinchi S, et al. Size of FLT3 internal tandem duplication has prognostic significance in patients with acute myeloid leukemia. Blood 2006;107(9): 3724–6.

[27] Schmid D, Heinze G, Linnerth B, et al. Prognostic significance of WT1 gene expression at diagnosis in adult de novo acute myeloid leukemia. Leukemia 1997;11(5):639–43.

[28] Barjesteh van Waalwijk van Doorn-Khosrovani S, Erpelinck C, Meijer J, et al. Biallelic mu-tations in the CEBPA gene and low CEBPA expression levels as prognostic markers in inter-mediate-risk AML. Hematol J 2003;4(1):31–40.

[29] Schnittger S, Kohl TM, Haferlach T, et al. KIT-D816 mutations in AML1-ETO-positive AML are associated with impaired event-free and overall survival. Blood 2006;107(5):1791–9.

[30] Suzuki T, Kiyoi H, Ozeki K, et al. Clinical characteristics and prognostic implications of NPM1 mutations in acute myeloid leukemia. Blood 2005;106(8):2854–61.

[31] Thiede C, Koch S, Creutzig E, et al. Prevalence and prognostic impact of NPM1 mutations in 1485 adult patients with acute myeloid leukemia (AML). Blood 2006;107(10):4011–20.

[32] Levis M, Allebach J, Tse KF, et al. A FLT3-targeted tyrosine kinase inhibitor is cytotoxic to leukemia cells in vitro and in vivo. Blood 2002;99(11):3885–91.

[33] Knapper S, Burnett AK, Littlewood T, et al. A phase 2 trial of the FLT3 inhibitor lestaurtinib (CEP701) as first-line treatment for older patients with acute myeloid leukemia not considered fit for intensive chemotherapy. Blood 2006;108(10):3262–70.

[34] Stirewalt DL, Radich JP. The role of FLT3 in haematopoietic malignancies. Nat Rev Cancer 2003;3(9):650–65.

[35] Druker BJ, Guilhot F, O'brien SG, et al. Five-year follow-up of patients receiving imatinib for chronic myeloid leukemia. N Engl J Med 2006;355(23):2408–17.

[36] Gorre ME, Mohammed M, Ellwood K, et al. Clinical resistance to STI-571 cancer therapy caused by BCR-ABL gene mutation or amplification. Science 2001;293(5531):876–80.

[37] Young MA, Shah NP, Chao LH, et al. Structure of the kinase domain of an imatinib-resistant Abl mutant in complex with the Aurora kinase inhibitor VX-680. Cancer Res 2006;66(2):1007–14.

[38] Kantarjian HM, Giles F, Gattermann N, et al. Nilotinib (formerly AMN107), a highly selective BCR-ABL tyrosine kinase inhibitor, is effective in patients with Philadelphia chromosome positive chronic myelogenous leukemia in chronic phase following imatinib resistance and intolerance. Blood 2007;110(10):3540–6.

[39] Mughal TI, Goldman JM. Emerging strategies for the treatment of mutant Bcr-Abl T315I myeloid leukemia. Clin Lymphoma Myeloma 2007;7(Suppl 2):S81–4.

[40] Kruglyak L, Nickerson DA. Variation is the spice of life. Nat Genet 2001;27(3):234–6.

[41] Feuk L, Carson AR, Scherer SW. Structural variation in the human genome. Nat Rev Genet 2006;7(2):85–97.

[42] Pandya U, Srivastava SK, Singhal SS, et al. Activity of allelic variants of Pi class human glutathione S-transferase toward chlorambucil. Biochem Biophys Res Commun 2000;278(1):258–62.

[43] Johansson AS, Stenberg G, Widersten M, et al. Structure-activity relationships and thermal stability of human glutathione transferase P1-1 governed by the H-site residue 105. J Mol Biol 1998;278(3):687–98.

[44] Stoehlmacher J, Park DJ, Zhang W, et al. Association between glutathione S-transferase P1, T1, and M1 genetic polymorphism and survival of patients with metastatic colorectal cancer. J Natl Cancer Inst 2002;94(12):936–42.

[45] Stoehlmacher J, Park DJ, Zhang W, et al. A multivariate analysis of genomic polymorphisms: prediction of clinical outcome to 5-FU/oxaliplatin combination chemotherapy in refractory colorectal cancer. Br J Cancer 2004;91(2):344–54.

[46] Dasgupta RK, Adamson PJ, Davies FE, et al. Polymorphic variation in GSTP1 modulates outcome following therapy for multiple myeloma. Blood 2003;102(7):2345–50.

[47] Goekkurt E, Hoehn S, Wolschke C, et al. Polymorphisms of glutathione S-transferases (GST) and thymidylate synthase (TS)–novel predictors for response and survival in gastric cancer patients. Br J Cancer 2006;94(2):281–6.

[48] Hohaus S, Di Ruscio A, Di Febo A, et al. Glutathione S-transferase P1 genotype and prognosis in Hodgkin's lymphoma. Clin Cancer Res 2005;11(6):2175–9.

[49] Sweeney C, McClure GY, Fares MY, et al. Association between survival after treatment for breast cancer and glutathione S-transferase P1 Ile105Val polymorphism. Cancer Res 2000;60(20):5621–4.

[50] Allan JM, Smith AG, Wheatley K, et al. Genetic variation in XPD predicts treatment outcome and risk of acute myeloid leukemia following chemotherapy. Blood 2004;104(13):3872–7.

[51] Fitzgibbon J, Smith LL, Raghavan M, et al. Association between acquired uniparental disomy and homozygous gene mutation in acute myeloid leukemias. Cancer Res 2005;65(20):9152–4.

[52] Raghavan M, Lillington DM, Skoulakis S, et al. Genome-wide single nucleotide polymorphism analysis reveals frequent partial uniparental disomy due to somatic recombination in acute myeloid leukemias. Cancer Res 2005;65(2):375–8.

[53] Strefford JC, van Delft FW, Robinson HM, et al. Complex genomic alterations and gene expression in acute lymphoblastic leukemia with intrachromosomal amplification of chromosome 21. Proc Natl Acad Sci U S A 2006;103(21):8167–72.

[54] Irving JA, Bloodworth L, Bown NP, et al. Loss of heterozygosity in childhood acute lymphoblastic leukemia detected by genome-wide microarray single nucleotide polymorphism analysis. Cancer Res 2005;65(8):3053–8.

[55] Hamblin TJ, Davis Z, Gardiner A, et al. Unmutated Ig V(H) genes are associated with a more aggressive form of chronic lymphocytic leukemia. Blood 1999;94(6):1848–54.

[56] Ardeshna KM, Smith P, Norton A, et al. Long-term effect of a watch and wait policy versus immediate systemic treatment for asymptomatic advanced-stage non-Hodgkin lymphoma: a randomised controlled trial. Lancet 2003;362(9383):516–22.

[57] Coulthard S, Hogarth L. The thiopurines: an update. Invest New Drugs 2005;23(6):523–32.

[58] Coulthard SA, Matheson EC, Hall AG, et al. The clinical impact of thiopurine methyltransferase polymorphisms on thiopurine treatment. Nucleosides Nucleotides Nucleic Acids 2004;23(8–9):1385–91.

[59] McLeod HL, Siva C. The thiopurine S-methyltransferase gene locus—implications for clinical pharmacogenomics. Pharmacogenomics 2002;3(1):89–98.

[60] Yates CR, Krynetski EY, Loennechen T, et al. Molecular diagnosis of thiopurine S-methyltransferase deficiency: genetic basis for azathioprine and mercaptopurine intolerance. Ann Intern Med 1997;126(8):608–14.

[61] Evans WE, Rodman J, Relling MV, et al. Individualized dosages of chemotherapy as a strategy to improve response for acute lymphocytic leukemia. Semin Hematol 1991;28(3 Suppl 4):15–21.

[62] McLeod HL, Miller DR, Evans WE. Azathioprine-induced myelosuppression in thiopurine methyltransferase deficient heart transplant recipient. Lancet 1993;341(8853):1151.

[63] van den Akker-van Marle ME, Gurwitz D, Detmar SB, et al. Cost-effectiveness of pharmacogenomics in clinical practice: a case study of thiopurine methyltransferase genotyping in acute lymphoblastic leukemia in Europe. Pharmacogenomics 2006;7(5):783–92.

[64] Tallman MS, Abutalib SA, Altman JK. The double hazard of thrombophilia and bleeding in acute promyelocytic leukemia. Semin Thromb Hemost 2007;33(4):330–8.

[65] Krejci O, Wunderlich M, Geiger H, et al. p53 signaling in response to increased DNA damage sensitizes AML1-ETO cells to stress-induced death. Blood 2008;111(4):2190–9.

[66] Park DJ, Stoehlmacher J, Zhang W, et al. A Xeroderma pigmentosum group D gene polymorphism predicts clinical outcome to platinum-based chemotherapy in patients with advanced colorectal cancer. Cancer Res 2001;61(24):8654–8.

[67] Wang D, Lippard SJ. Cellular processing of platinum anticancer drugs. Nat Rev Drug Discov 2005;4(4):307–20.

[68] Mehta PA, Alonzo TA, Gerbing RB, et al. XPD Lys751Gln polymorphism in the etiology and outcome of childhood acute myeloid leukemia: a Children's Oncology Group report. Blood 2006;107(1):39–45.

[69] Kuptsova N, Kopecky KJ, Godwin J, et al. Polymorphisms in DNA repair genes and therapeutic outcomes of AML patients from SWOG clinical trials. Blood 2007;109(9):3936–44.

[70] Francis S, Karanth M, Pratt G, et al. The effect of immunoglobulin VH gene mutation status and other prognostic factors on the incidence of major infections in patients with chronic lymphocytic leukemia. Cancer 2006;107(5):1023–33.

[71] Mackall CL. T-cell immunodeficiency following cytotoxic antineoplastic therapy: a review. Stem Cells 2000;18(1):10–8.

[72] Allan JM, Wild CP, Rollinson S, et al. Polymorphism in glutathione S-transferase P1 is associated with susceptibility to chemotherapy-induced leukemia. Proc Natl Acad Sci U S A 2001;98(20):11592–7.

[73] Allan JM, Rabkin CS. Genetic susceptibility to iatrogenic malignancy. Pharmacogenomics 2005;6(6):615–28.

Second Primary Cancers: An Overview

Andrea K. Ng, MD, MPH[a],*, Lois B. Travis, MD, ScD[b]

[a]Department of Radiation Oncology, Dana-Farber Cancer Institute, Brigham and Women's Hospital, Harvard Medical School, 75 Francis Street, ASB1-L2, Boston, MA 02115, USA
[b]Division of Cancer Epidemiology and Genetics, National Cancer Institute, Department of Health and Human Services, National Institutes of Health, Bethesda, MD 20892, USA

S ubstantial improvements in the last few decades in cancer detection and supportive care along with advances in therapy have led to growing numbers of cancer survivors. In 2004, there were an estimated 10.7 million cancer survivors in the United States [1], with an overall 5-year relative survival rate of almost 66% [1]. In view of the prolongation of survival in increasing numbers of patients [2], identification and quantification of the late effects of cancer and its therapy have become critical. One of the most serious events experienced by cancer survivors is the diagnosis of a new cancer. The number of patients who have second or higher-order cancers is growing rapidly, with independent malignancies composing about 16% (or 1 in 6) incident cancers reported to the National Cancer Institute's (NCI's) Surveillance, Epidemiology, and End Results (SEER) program in 2004 [1]. Further, solid tumors are a primary cause of mortality among several populations of long-term survivors, including patients who have Hodgkin lymphoma (HL) [3]. Second cancers can be attributable to the late effects of therapy, the influence of lifestyle choices (eg, tobacco or alcohol use), host determinants, environmental exposures, and combinations of effects, including gene–environment and gene–gene interactions [4]. Elevated risks for subsequent malignancies in cancer survivors may also result from closer follow-up by health care providers. Travis and colleagues [5] recently categorized second primary cancers into three major groups according to dominant etiologic factors (ie, treatment-related, syndromic, and those attributable to shared etiologic influences) underscoring the non-exclusivity of these delineations. The focus of this article is treatment-associated malignancies in survivors of selected adult cancers, particularly those for whom a large amount of data has accrued. Second malignant neoplasms after childhood cancer are reviewed elsewhere in this issue by Hudson and colleagues. The follow-up of childhood cancer survivors in this issue. The reader is referred elsewhere for comprehensive reviews of multiple primary cancers [4,6] and discussions of possible underlying genetic mechanisms [5,7].

*Corresponding author. E-mail address: ang@lroc.harvard.edu (A.K. Ng).

0889-8588/08/$ – see front matter
doi:10.1016/j.hoc.2008.01.007

SECOND MALIGNANCIES AFTER SPECIFIC TYPES OF CANCER

Hodgkin Lymphoma

The largest body of literature on second malignancies exists for survivors of HL, because of the high curability of the disease, the relatively young age at diagnosis, and the resultant long life expectancy. Treatment-related leukemias in patients who had HL were first described in the early 1970s [8], with the risk highest in the first 10 years after treatment [9–13]. It later became apparent that the risk was largely related to the use of alkylating chemotherapy, with evidence for a strong dose–response relationship [11,14]. Splenectomy and the addition of radiation therapy to chemotherapy have also been implicated as risk factors, although the data are not consistent [10,15]. The prognosis of patients who have HL who develop leukemia is extremely poor, with a median survival of less than 1 year [16]. Given the replacement of mechlorethamine, vincristine, procarbazine, and prednisone (MOPP) with Adriamycin, bleomycin, vinblastine, and dacarbazine (ABVD), the risk for leukemia has been substantially reduced. Leukemogenic agents are still often used in the setting of salvage therapy, however, and are present in some of the newer regimens, including bleomycin, etoposide, Adriamycin, cyclophosphamide, procarbazine, and prednisone (BEACOPP) [17]. The risk for leukemia may therefore persist in subgroups of Hodgkin lymphoma treated with modern therapy.

An increased risk for non-Hodgkin's lymphoma (NHL) after HL has also been observed [18], although the timing and relationship with prior therapy is unclear. Patients who have history of lymphocyte-predominant HL have been shown to be at higher risk for developing NHL than those who have other histologic types. The prognosis of NHL after HL seems to be comparable to patients who have de novo advanced-stage NHL [18].

As the number of survivors of HL has increased and with longer follow-up time, solid tumors have emerged as the major subtype of second malignancy, accounting for up to 75% to 80% of all cases [19–21]. Radiotherapy-associated solid tumors typically develop after a long latency (typically at least 5 to 9 years) from initial treatment of HL. In addition, the risk seems to persist as long as 30 years [21]. The contribution of radiation therapy to the development of solid tumors after Hodgkin lymphoma is supported by the observation that most of the solid tumors arise within or at the edges of prior radiation treatment fields. In addition, more recent studies showed a significant radiation dose–response relationship in the development of specific types of solid tumors after HL. In a large international case-control study of young women who had HL who developed breast cancer (105 cases; 266 matched controls), radiation dose to the area of the breast where the tumor developed in the case (and a comparable area in matched controls) was estimated for each case-control set [22]. Breast cancer risk increased significantly with increasing radiation dose to reach eightfold for the highest dose category (median dose 42 Gy) compared with the lowest dose group (<4 Gy) (P trend < .001). In a separate Dutch study [23], similar results were found, with most of the latter patients also included in the international effort [22]. In both studies [22,23], patients who received both chemotherapy and radiation therapy had a significantly decreased risk (about half) compared with those treated with radiation therapy alone, and the radiation-related risks were attenuated by treatment with alkylating agents or a radiation dose of 5 Gy or more delivered to the ovaries. The Dutch study clearly showed that the substantial risk reduction associated with chemotherapy was attributable to the high frequency of premature menopause in chemotherapy-treated patients. Results of both studies showed that ovarian hormones are a crucial factor to promote tumorigenesis once radiation has produced an initiating event [22,23].

A significant dose–response relationship with radiation has similarly been demonstrated for the development of lung cancer after HL. In a study by Travis and colleagues [24] using patients who received less than 5 Gy to the area of the lung in which cancer developed as the reference group, the risk for lung cancer increased with increasing radiation dose to the area of the lung in which cancer developed, even among patients who received 40 or more Gy (P trend with dose $< .001$); risk reached seven to ninefold at doses of 30 or more Gy.

The data on solid tumors after radiation therapy for HL were based on patients treated when large treatment fields and higher radiation doses were typically used. The radiation treatment field is significantly smaller with the current standard of involved-field radiation therapy as part of combined modality therapy. Efforts are also ongoing to explore additional reductions in radiation dose. More recently, there is a trend toward involved-node radiation therapy that further reduces the exposure of normal tissue to radiation [25]. It is thus expected that patients who receive radiation therapy in the modern era face a lower risk for second malignancy.

There is a paucity of long-term data on HL patients treated with chemotherapy alone because of the historically prominent role of radiation therapy in the cure of this disease. Most studies do not have large enough numbers of patients who have HL treated with chemotherapy alone and with sufficient follow-up time to meaningfully examine the long-term risk for solid tumors. In a collaborative British cohort study of 1693 patients who had HL treated with chemotherapy alone, the relative risk (RR) for lung cancer was significantly increased (RR = 3.3; 95% CI, 2.2–4.7) [26]. This increased risk was comparable in magnitude to HL patients who received either radiation therapy alone (RR = 2.9; 95% CI, 1.9–4.1) or combined modality therapy (RR = 4.3; 95% CI, 2.9–6.2). Most patients in this study were treated with alkylating agent–based chemotherapy. The significance of alkylating agent in subsequent lung cancer development after HL was confirmed in a case-control study by the same group [27] and in the NCI international case-control study described previously [24] with both investigations showing a significant dose–response relationship between cumulative dose of alkylating agent chemotherapy and lung cancer risk.

Several other factors have been shown to influence the risk for treatment-related second malignancy after HL. Young age at mantle irradiation has consistently been shown to be associated with significantly increased risk for breast cancer in women [16,21,22,28]. In a recent population-based cohort study by Hodgson and colleagues [21], the absolute risks for breast cancer in women diagnosed with HL at ages 15 to 25 were 34 to 47 per 10,000 person years at 10 years, which was higher than the absolute risks for women in the general population between 50 and 54 years, a typical age when mammography screening is recommended.

Increasing awareness of the large risk for breast cancer following therapy for HL at a young age has created the need for informed counseling. Estimates of the cumulative absolute risk for breast cancer among young women treated for HL at age 30 years or younger have been sparse and inconsistent, however, spanning 4.2% to 34% at 20 to 25 years after therapy [26,29–31]. Most estimates have not taken into account the influence of alkylating agent therapy, which can lower breast cancer risk [22,23], or the effect of competing causes of mortality [32]. Accurate projections of breast cancer risk, as available for women in the general population [33], are important to evaluate the disease burden among the growing population of HL survivors treated with regimens of the past and to facilitate the development of risk-adapted long-term follow-up recommendations. Estimates of the cumulative absolute risk for breast cancer among women treated for HL at age 30 years or younger were recently provided in measures of radiation dose and chemotherapy, which are available from medical records [34]. The estimates also took into account age and calendar year of HL diagnosis, age at counseling, baseline breast cancer incidence rates, and competing causes of mortality. For example, for an HL survivor who was treated at age 25 years with a chest radiation dose of at least 40 Gy without alkylating agents, estimated cumulative absolute risks for breast cancer by age 35, 45, and 55 years were 1.4%, 11.1%, and 29.0%, respectively. Cumulative absolute risks were lower in women also treated with alkylating agents. In comparison, in the general population the absolute risks for breast cancer in white women from age 20 years to ages 30, 40, 50, and 60 years are, respectively, 0.04%, 0.5%, 2.0%, and 4.3%. The researchers [34] cautioned that the risk estimates are most relevant for HL survivors treated with past regimens, and should be used with considerable caution in patients treated with more recent approaches described previously, including limited-field radiotherapy or ovary-sparing chemotherapy.

Tobacco exposure is another important factor that influences the treatment-related risk for lung cancer among HL survivors. In a case-control study by Travis and colleagues [24], in which the reference group consisted of patients who had HL who had minimal radiation exposure and who were nonsmokers or light smokers, those patients who received either alkylating agent chemotherapy alone or 5 Gy or more of radiation therapy alone to the area of the lung in which cancer developed later experienced 4.3-fold and 7.2-fold increased risks for lung cancer, respectively. The relative risks increased to 16.8-fold and 20.2-fold, respectively, in those patients who also smoked at least one pack of cigarettes per day. For cigarette smokers (at least one pack per day) who had also received alkylating chemotherapy and 5 Gy or more of radiation therapy to the area of the lung in which cancer developed, the relative risk for subsequent lung cancer was 49.1, consistent with a multiplicative effect of smoking history on the risk for treatment-related lung cancer.

As our knowledge of second malignancy risk after HL therapy accumulates, increasing research and clinical efforts have been directed toward addressing this important problem, including the development of programs for early detection and prevention of a new malignancy, risk factor modification, and initial treatment modification and reduction [35]. These efforts may serve as a model for managing survivors of other primary cancers for whom long-term data on excess second malignancies are only now emerging.

Non-Hodgkin Lymphoma

Compared to survivors of HL, the data on second malignancy after treatment of NHL is less extensive, and the documented excess risk seems less pronounced. This observation may be attributable to the heterogeneity of the disease and lower cure rate in subsets of patients, the diverse treatment options, or the older age of patients at diagnosis (and the larger baseline risk for cancer). Among several large population-based studies on survivors of NHL, an excess risk for leukemia, HL, lung cancer, head and neck cancer, bladder cancer, cutaneous melanoma, Kaposi sarcoma, and mesothelioma have been observed [36–44].

Unlike HL, the effect of chemotherapy on second malignancy risk, including risk for solid tumors, seems to be more apparent in NHL survivors. In a case-control study by Travis and colleagues [45] focusing on genitourinary cancer after NHL, exposure to cyclophosphamide was associated with a significantly increased risk for bladder cancer compared with patients who did not received this cytotoxic drug (RR = 4.5; 95% CI, 1.6–13.6) (P trend for cumulative dose < .001). The doses of cyclophosphamide associated with increased bladder cancer risk in this study, however, were considerably higher than what is currently used in standard-dose therapy.

The EORTC reported on the risk for second malignancy in 2837 patients who had NHL treated with the ACVBP regimen [36]. Only 4.3% of patients in this cohort received radiation therapy. The relative risk for leukemia was 5.65 ($P = .006$) among male survivors and 19.9 ($P < .001$) among female survivors when compared with the normal, matched population. The relative risk for lung cancer was also significantly increased among men (RR = 2.45; $P < .001$). In another large retrospective cohort study conducted by the British Collaborative Group, the risk for second malignancy among 2456 patients who had NHL was examined [37]. Among the 1274 patients treated with chemotherapy alone (consisting mostly of cyclophosphamide, doxorubicin, vincristine, and prednisone) significantly increased relative risks for leukemia, colorectal cancer, and lung cancer were seen (risks of 10.5 [$P<.001$], 2.1 [$P<.05$], and 1.9 [$P<.01$], respectively.) Exposure to chemotherapy alone may thus be associated with an increased risk for not only leukemia but also selected solid tumors in patients who have NHL, although analytic studies are required to confirm these observations.

Although radiation therapy may increase the risk for several specific types of solid tumors after NHL, including bladder cancer [45] and bone sarcoma, its impact on the overall risk for second malignancies is less certain. For instance, in the British Collaborative study, although the relative risks for lung cancer and colorectal cancer were significantly increased, the relative risk for all solid tumors was not significantly increased after chemotherapy alone (RR = 1.0; 95% CI, 0.7%–1.4%) [37]. The addition of radiation therapy to chemotherapy also did not lead to an increased relative risk for solid malignancy (RR = 1.2; 95% CI, 0.8%–1.7%). In a population-based cohort study using data from the SEER program for 77,823 patients who had NHL, similar findings were observed in that no significant difference in relative risks for second malignancy was found between unirradiated and irradiated patients (RR = 1.13; 95% CI, 1.1–1.17 versus RR = 1.18; 95% CI, 1.12–1.23) [38]. Further, in several retrospective and prospective studies that reported on long-term second malignancy risk after radiation therapy for NHL, most of these second cancers were found to arise outside of the radiation field [36,46,47].

Testicular Cancer

Testicular cancer and HL have several similar characteristics, in that both are highly curable and typically affect young individuals who have a life expectancy close to that of the normal population after treatment completion. Historically, treatment also included the use of relatively large radiation therapy fields. As in patients who had HL, second malignancy is an important cause of death among survivors of testicular cancer [48,49].

The types of second malignancy documented in survivors of testicular cancer include leukemia and several solid tumors, including mesothelioma, cancers of the lung, thyroid, esophagus, stomach, pancreas, colon, rectum, kidney, bladder, and connective tissue [50]. An excess risk for contralateral testicular cancer has also been observed, which is likely related to underlying predisposition rather than prior treatment. In a large population-based study of 29,515 men who had a history of testicular cancer, the 15-year cumulative risk for contralateral testicular cancer was 1.9%, which was 12.4-fold higher than that expected in the normal population [51].

For the remaining solid tumors, depending on the sites of development, they are likely in part a reflection of the historical routine use of para-aortic and pelvic radiation therapy, and earlier on, the use of mediastinal irradiation in patients who had testicular cancer. In the largest cohort study on testicular cancer survivors to date, using international population-based data, Travis and colleagues [50] reported on the solid tumor risk among 40,576 patients. At a mean follow-up of 11.8 years, the relative risks for developing a solid tumor were significantly increased after radiation therapy alone and chemotherapy alone (RR of 2.0 and 1.8, respectively). The relative risk was higher among patients who received both chemotherapy and radiation therapy

(RR = 2.9), although it was not statistically significantly higher than the risk associated with single-modality therapy. For solid tumors that were likely related to prior radiation treatment based on the sites of development, the relative risks increased with increasing follow-up time.

The risk for leukemia after testicular cancer has been shown to be related to both chemotherapy and radiation therapy [49,52–54]. Chemotherapeutic agents that have been associated with the development of leukemia include cisplatin and etoposide [52–54]. A population-based study by Travis and colleagues [52] explored treatment-associated leukemia in 18,567 men who had testicular cancer who had survived at least 1 year. The risk for leukemia increased significantly with increasing radiation field size, which was reflected in dose to active bone marrow. In addition, after taking into account the amount of radiation exposure to active bone marrow, the risk for leukemia was also significantly associated with cumulative dose of cisplatin received.

Breast Cancer

Among the various types of second cancers observed in survivors of breast cancer, the largest amount of data exists for contralateral breast cancer, which is related in large part to pre-existing breast cancer risk factors [55–59]. Prior radiation therapy may also contribute to the risk, especially among women who received treatment at a young age. Another malignancy after breast cancer that is related to underlying predisposition and to previous breast cancer therapy, particularly tamoxifen therapy, is endometrial cancer. Lung cancer and sarcoma are other solid tumors that have been reported in breast cancer survivors, with risks largely related to exposure to radiation therapy. An increased risk for leukemia after breast cancer has also been observed, which is associated with exposure to both chemotherapy and radiation therapy.

The risk for contralateral breast cancer is increased two to fivefold among patients who have breast cancer [58]. Conflicting data exist on the contribution of radiation therapy to the excess risk [55,56,58,60]. In a case-control study by Boice and colleagues [58], the overall relative risk for contralateral breast cancer was not significantly increased after radiation therapy (RR = 1.19; 95% CI, 0.94–1.15). Among women who were younger than 45 years of age at the time of irradiation, however, the relative risk was significantly elevated at 1.59 (95% CI, 1.07–2.36). In the Early Breast Cancer Trialists' Collaborative Group report, which evaluated the effects of radiotherapy, a significantly increased risk for contralateral breast cancer was found, mainly during the period 5 to14 years after randomization (RR = 1.43; P = .00001), and the increased risk associated with radiation therapy was significant even among women aged 50 years or older when randomized (RR = 1.25; P = .002) [61]. In contrast, in another large case-control study from Denmark, there was no significant difference in the risk for contralateral breast cancer in women who did and did not receive radiation therapy, regardless of age at treatment [59]. In the Danish study, it was found that the second breast cancers were evenly distributed in the medial, lateral, and central portions of the breast, which also argued against a causal role of radiotherapy in tumorigenesis. A recent large-scale, single-institution study from Institut Curie which included 13,472 women, similarly failed to show an increased risk for contralateral breast cancer when comparing women who did or did not receive radiation therapy (RR = 1.1; 95% CI, 0.96–1.27). Analysis by age, however, was not performed in that study [55].

Tamoxifen is used in many women who have estrogen receptor–positive breast cancer as adjuvant therapy, and has been shown to reduce the risk for contralateral breast cancer by 30% to 40% [62]. On the other hand, several large studies have clearly demonstrated a two to fourfold increased risk for endometrial cancer after tamoxifen therapy [63,64]. Earlier studies indicated that endometrial cancer after tamoxifen may have a more favorable prognosis, although recent data have raised the concern that tamoxifen-related endometrial cancers may have a more aggressive behavior [65–67]. Most cases are detected at an early stage and are amenable to surgical resection, however. Endometrial cancer after tamoxifen therapy therefore does not seem to be associated with poorer endometrial cancer–specific survival.

Radiation therapy is an important modality in the treatment of breast cancer, either as part of breast-conserving therapy or as postmastectomy radiation therapy. Other than contralateral breast cancer, which may be related to prior radiation therapy, several other solid tumors have also been linked to a history of radiation therapy for breast cancer. These include lung cancer, soft tissue sarcoma, and esophageal cancer.

In several studies [55,68,69], women who received radiation therapy have been shown to be at a 1.5 to threefold increased risk for developing lung cancer compared with women who did not receive radiation therapy. The increased risk seemed to be more clearly related to postmastectomy radiation therapy, in which the radiation target volume often also include the supraclavicular, axillary, or internal mammary nodal region, thus exposing a larger volume of underlying lung tissue to the radiation, whereas the risk after post-lumpectomy radiation therapy is less certain [70,71]. The observation that lung cancer after breast cancer therapy is more frequently found in the ipsilateral lung also supports the contributing role of radiation therapy to the risk [70]. Several studies showed further increase in the risk for lung cancer among smokers who have received breast irradiation [72,73], although the interaction between tobacco exposure and prior radiation therapy on subsequent lung cancer risk is not as well elucidated as in survivors of HL.

Although the occurrence of sarcoma after breast cancer is a rare event, with a 15-year incidence rate of less than 0.5%, the relative risk has been estimated to be as high as 7, because of the low background incidence in the general population [55,74–76]. In a study by Rubino and colleagues [77], all observed sarcomas occurred among women who had initially received radiation therapy, and in all cases the sarcomas were located in the irradiated fields or in the upper extremity of the arm ipsilateral to the treated breast. Further, a significant dose–response relationship was demonstrated. By estimating the initial radiation dose to the site of sarcoma development, using a dose of 14 Gy or less to the site as reference, women who received 14 to 44 Gy had a 1.6-fold increased risk for sarcoma, whereas those who received 45 Gy or more to the site had a 30.6-fold increased risk ($P < .001$). Angiosarcoma as a malignancy after breast cancer was initially shown to be associated with chronic lymphedema following radical mastectomy [78]. With the increasing use of radiation therapy, there have been a growing number of reports of cutaneous angiosarcoma of the breast arising in the radiation field [76,79–81]. Unlike other radiation-related soft tissue sarcoma, angiosarcoma has a short latency and can occur in the first 5 years after therapy.

The increased risk for leukemia following breast cancer is related to prior chemotherapy and radiation therapy [82–85]. In a case-control study by Curtis and colleagues [82] of women treated for breast cancer between 1973 and 1985, 90 women who developed leukemia and 264 matched controls were studied. Compared with women who did not receive alkylating chemotherapy or radiation therapy, the relative risk for acute myelogenous leukemia after radiation therapy alone, alkylating chemotherapy alone, and both chemotherapy and radiation therapy were 2.4, 10.0, and 17.4, respectively. A significant dose–response effect was observed for either cumulative dose of melphalan, cyclophosphamide, or radiation to the active bone marrow, and the subsequent risk for leukemia. This study was conducted in an era when higher cumulative doses of chemotherapy and larger field radiation therapy were used, however. Melphalan-containing regimens are also no longer used in the treatment of breast cancer. Recent data showed that the risk for acute leukemia is more significantly associated with dose intensity of cyclophosphamide rather than cumulative dose of chemotherapy [86], a finding that is of relevance with the increasing trend toward use of dose-intensified regimens for breast cancer.

In addition to evolving systemic therapy for breast cancer treatment, which may affect the subsequent second malignancy risk, recent advances in radiation therapy, including use of intensity modulated therapy radiation (IMRT), and the growing interest in partial breast irradiation [87], may also alter the second malignancy risk profile of breast cancer survivors. The risks associated with these newer radiation therapy approaches and techniques remain to be clarified.

Prostate Cancer

In recent years, there has been increasing attention to the risk for second malignancies after radiation therapy for prostate cancer [88–95]. Neugut and colleagues [95] were the first to report on the effect of radiotherapy for prostate carcinoma on the risk for second cancers in a population-based study using data from the SEER program. Men who received radiation therapy had a significantly increased risk for developing bladder cancer after a latent period of 8 years (RR = 1.5; 95% CI, 1.1–2.0), whereas the risk was not increased among men who did not receive radiation therapy. In a more recent study based on the Mayo Clinic Cancer Registry [91], whereas the overall relative risk for bladder cancer after radiation therapy was not significantly increased, among the subset of patients who received adjuvant radiation therapy after a radical prostatectomy the relative risk for bladder cancer was fivefold higher than expected ($P = .05$), which may be because of the larger volume of bladder exposed to the radiation in the postoperative setting.

In the study by Neugut and colleagues, an increased risk for rectal cancer or leukemia after radiation therapy was not seen. In a subsequent study by Brenner and colleagues [94], which also used data from the SEER program, men who were treated initially with radiation therapy were compared with men treated with surgery alone. Patients who received radiation therapy had a significantly increased risk for bladder cancer, rectal cancer, sarcoma, and lung cancer. The finding of a significant association between irradiation for prostate cancer and lung cancer risk was attributed to low scatter doses of radiation to the lungs. This observation may be more pertinent in patients who received cobalt irradiation to the whole pelvis. A more recent study using the linked SEER-Medicare database contained a larger number of patients, including those treated in the more recent era [89]. Men who received external beam radiation therapy had a statistically significantly increased risk for developing cancers of the bladder, rectum, colon, brain, stomach, and lung, and melanoma, with odds ratios ranging from 1.25 to 1.85, when compared with men who did not receive external beam radiation therapy. Patients who received radioactive implants with or without external beam radiation therapy, however, did not have a significantly increased risk for second cancer when compared with the no radiation therapy cohort.

In a study from the British Columbia Tumor Registry [93], among patients who received radiation therapy, significantly elevated risks for colorectal cancer (RR = 1.21; $P < .01$), pleural cancer (RR = 2.28; $P < .01$) and sarcoma (RR = 1.7; $P < .05$) were observed. Although the bladder cancer risk was not significantly increased in the radiation therapy cohort, the risks for bladder cancer (RR = 1.32; $P < .01$) and testicular cancer (RR = 2.82; $P < .05$) were significantly increased in the non-irradiation cohort, which was believed to be related to heightened surveillance.

Another recent report also based on data from the SEER program focused on the risk for rectal cancer after prostatic irradiation [90]. Unlike previous studies, a significant association between radiation therapy and a subsequently increased risk for rectal cancer was not found. Results of Cox proportional hazards analysis (with prostate irradiation, prostate surgery, and age at diagnosis entered as covariates) showed that only age was associated with an increased risk for subsequent rectal cancer.

Most studies on malignancies after prostate cancer therapy used data from population-based registries. The conflicting findings on the contribution of radiation therapy to various second malignancies after prostate cancer may be because most registries collect data only on initial course of therapy, registration of initial treatment is incomplete in some registries, and selection criteria differ for patients given surgery versus radiation therapy; moreover, given the limited data available in most population-based registries, it is not possible to identify or to control for confounding factors. Patients who have significant comorbid illnesses or heavy smoking histories may not be selected for surgery and may be more likely to undergo radiation therapy. Further, among patients who received radiation therapy, treatment-related effects, including proctitis, rectal bleeding, cystitis, and hematuria may lead to additional colonoscopies or cystoscopies, which in turn can result in an apparent increased incidence of colorectal or other urologic cancers.

In studies that demonstrate a significant risk for cancers after radiation therapy for prostate cancer, the overall incidence seems to be low. In the study by Brenner and colleagues that included patients who received larger-field cobalt irradiation, the risk for developing a radiation-associated second malignancy was estimated at 1 in 290 [94]. In the last several years, IMR has been increasingly adopted in the treatment of prostate cancer to allow more conformal dose distribution and dose escalation [96]. Depending on treatment energy, IMRT is associated with a three to fivefold higher number of monitor units as compared with conventional treatment. Using the National Council of Radiation Protection and Measurements risk coefficients for specific anatomic sites, the risk for second malignancy using IMRT techniques has been estimated to be two to three times higher than that after conventional radiation therapy [97]. These estimates are yet to be confirmed in epidemiologic studies with sufficient follow-up time for patients who have received IMRT.

Cervical Cancer

Survivors of cervical cancer are at increased risk for developing several second malignancies, some of which can be explained by shared infectious cause or environmental risk factors, whereas others are attributable to previous treatment exposures. Kleinerman and colleagues [98] were among the first to report on the risk for second malignancy following cervical cancer. Compared with the general population, survivors of cervical cancer had a 1.4-fold increased risk for a second malignancy. A history of radiation therapy was associated with a significantly increased risk for several cancers in the pelvic radiation field, including tumors of bladder, kidney, rectum, corpus uteri, and ovary. Since then, several studies have confirmed these findings [99–101]. Chaturvedi and colleagues [102] recently updated and expanded these data based on 104,760 1-year survivors of cervical cancer reported to 13 population-based cancer registries in Denmark, Finland, Norway, Sweden, and the United States. In this larger study with longer follow-up time, a significantly elevated relative risk (RR = 1.3; 95% CI, 1.28–1.33) for second malignancy was again found. Moreover, the authors showed that following radiation therapy for cervical cancer, the risks for second cancers of the rectum/anus, colon, urinary bladder, ovary, and other female genital sites remained significantly elevated for more than 40 years. Several second cancers were likely related to shared etiologic factors rather than radiation therapy, because an increased risk was also observed among the non–radiation therapy cohort. These included cancers of the pharynx, genital sites, and rectum/anus, which are related to human papillomavirus infections; and cancers of the lungs, pancreas, and urinary bladder, which are related to tobacco use. In this study, younger age at cervical cancer treatment was associated with a significantly higher cumulative risk for second cancer.

In the last decade there has been increasing use of concurrent platinum-based chemotherapy with radiation therapy for the treatment of cervical cancer [103–105], which has been associated with significantly improved treatment outcome. As more women are cured of their disease, whether chemotherapy might contribute to the risk for second malignancies following cervical cancer should be explored. The persistence of platinum-DNA adducts in numerous human tissues long after treatment has been completed [106], albeit observed at higher doses of platinum-based chemotherapy, heightens the concern about late effects. Further, platinum causes solid tumors and leukemia in laboratory animals [107]. A statistically significant relation between increasing cumulative dose of platinum and increasing leukemia risk has been reported in survivors of testicular cancer [52] and ovarian cancer [108].

Head and Neck

Approximately 15% to 20% of patients previously treated for head and neck malignancies will be diagnosed with a second tumor, with the most common sites being another head and neck site, lung, or esophagus [109]. The increased risk for a second malignancy in patients who have head and neck cancer is largely related to exposure to tobacco and alcohol. Individual susceptibility to the mutagenic effect of carcinogens may also contribute to the risk [110]. In contrast with the other primary cancers discussed previously, treatment does not seem to play a clear causal role.

Several lines of evidence support the hypothesis that second malignancies in patients who have head and neck cancer are largely related to shared risk factors. These include: (1) the constant annual risk of 2% to 5% after a primary head and neck cancer, without any indication of a requisite latency period [111], (2) the observation that lung cancer is more commonly seen after laryngeal cancer, both of which are related to smoking, whereas esophageal cancer is more commonly seen after pharyngeal cancer, which is related to alcohol use and smoking [111–113], (3) the lack of an increase in second malignancy risk after cancers of the nasal cavity, paranasal sinuses, and nasopharynx, disease sites that are not related to tobacco and alcohol history [114], and (4) findings of a dose-dependent relationship between the amount of tobacco and alcohol use and the risk for second tumor development [111,112,115].

In addition to environmental factors, genetic factors may also modify the risk for second malignancies in patients who have head and neck cancer. In one study, relatives of patients who had a history of multiple head and neck cancers were at significantly higher risk for developing an upper aerodigestive cancer than relatives of patients who had only a single head and neck cancer (8.9% versus 2.5%, $P < .00001$). In addition, having one or more relatives who had a respiratory or upper digestive tract cancer was associated with a significantly higher risk for second cancers among patients who had head and neck cancer (odds ratio, 3.8; 95% CI, 2.0–7.6) [116]. These findings suggest that, in addition to external carcinogens, genetic susceptibility may influence the risk for the development of second malignancies in patients who have head and neck cancers.

Because of the high risk for second malignancies involving the aerodigestive tract, investigators have explored the use of chemoprevention in this population [117,118], although no clear beneficial effects have been demonstrated to date. In the meantime, smoking cessation is the most effective intervention for the prevention of second tumors in this high-risk population.

SUMMARY

As increasing numbers of patients who have cancer are cured, the emergence of second malignant neoplasms has emerged as a significant problem that can limit long-term survival and quality of life. Efforts to quantify and characterize the risks for second malignancies have important implications for patient counseling, behavioral changes, screening, and prevention strategies among cancer survivors. Whenever effective screening methods (eg, mammographic examination) are available, these should be included in patient follow-up. Preventive strategies (eg, smoking cessation, avoidance of ultraviolet light) may also diminish the risk for selected second cancers, and cancer survivors should be encouraged to adopt practices consistent with a healthy lifestyle. An improved understanding of therapy-related second malignancies can guide alterations in regimens to minimize cytotoxic treatment exposure. Modification or reduction of existing treatments that have proven and established efficacy, however, should not be conducted outside the setting of clinical trials. Moreover, it is important to keep in mind that second malignancies, although serious sequelae, are not seen unless a patient survives a cancer diagnosis. The survival benefits provided by many cancer treatments thus greatly outweigh the risk for developing a second primary cancer.

References

[1] Ries L, Melbert D, Krapcho M, et al. SEER cancer statistics review, 1975–2004. Bethesda (MA): National Cancer Institute; 2007.

[2] Cancer survivors: living longer, and now, better. Lancet 2004;364:2153–4.

[3] Dores G, Schonfeld S, Chen J, et al. Long-term cause-specific mortality among 41–146 one-year survivors of Hodgkin lymphoma (HL). Acta Oncologica 2005;23:562S.

[4] Travis LB. Therapy-associated solid tumors. Acta Oncol 2002;41:323–33.

[5] Travis LB, Rabkin CS, Brown LM, et al. Cancer survivorship—genetic susceptibility and second primary cancers: research strategies and recommendations. J Natl Cancer Inst 2006;98:15–25.

[6] van Leeuwen FE, Travis LB. Second cancers. In: DeVita VT, Hellman S, Rosenberg SA, et al, editors. Cancer: principles and practice of oncology. 7th edition. Philadelphia: Lippincott Williams & Wilkins; 2005. p. 2575–602.

[7] Allan JM, Travis LB. Mechanisms of therapy-related carcinogenesis. Nat Rev Cancer 2005;5:943–55.

[8] Arseneau JC, Sponzo RW, Levin DL, et al. Nonlymphomatous malignant tumors complicating Hodgkin's disease. Possible association with intensive therapy. N Engl J Med 1972;287:1119–22.

[9] Cimino G, Papa G, Tura S, et al. Second primary cancer following Hodgkin's disease: updated results of an Italian multicentric study. J Clin Oncol 1991;9:432–7.

[10] Henry-Amar M. Second cancer after the treatment for Hodgkin's disease: a report from the International Database on Hodgkin's Disease. Ann Oncol 1992;3(Suppl 4):117–28.

[11] Kaldor JM, Day NE, Clarke EA, et al. Leukemia following Hodgkin's disease. N Engl J Med 1990;322:7–13.

[12] Tucker MA, Coleman CN, Cox RS, et al. Risk of second cancers after treatment for Hodgkin's disease. N Engl J Med 1988;318:76–81.

[13] Valagussa P, Santoro A, Fossati-Bellani F, et al. Second acute leukemia and other malignancies following treatment for Hodgkin's disease. J Clin Oncol 1986;4:830–7.

[14] van Leeuwen FE, Chorus AM, van den Belt-Dusebout AW, et al. Leukemia risk following Hodgkin's disease: relation to cumulative dose of alkylating agents, treatment with teniposide combinations, number of episodes of chemotherapy, and bone marrow damage. J Clin Oncol 1994;12:1063–73.

[15] Andrieu JM, Ifrah N, Payen C, et al. Increased risk of secondary acute nonlymphocytic leukemia after extended-field radiation therapy combined with MOPP chemotherapy for Hodgkin's disease. J Clin Oncol 1990;8:1148–54.

[16] Ng AK, Bernardo MV, Weller E, et al. Second malignancy after Hodgkin disease treated with radiation therapy with or without chemotherapy: long-term risks and risk factors. Blood 2002;100:1989–96.

[17] Diehl V, Franklin J, Pfreundschuh M, et al. Standard and increased-dose BEACOPP chemotherapy compared with COPP-ABVD for advanced Hodgkin's disease. N Engl J Med 2003;348:2386–95.

[18] Rueffer U, Josting A, Franklin J, et al. Non-Hodgkin's lymphoma after primary Hodgkin's disease in the German Hodgkin's Lymphoma Study Group: incidence, treatment, and prognosis. J Clin Oncol 2001;19:2026–32.

[19] Biti G, Cellai E, Magrini SM, et al. Second solid tumors and leukemia after treatment for Hodgkin's disease: an analysis of 1121 patients from a single institution. Int J Radiat Oncol Biol Phys 1994;29:25–31.

[20] Doria R, Holford T, Farber LR, et al. Second solid malignancies after combined modality therapy for Hodgkin's disease. J Clin Oncol 1995;13:2016–22.

[21] Hodgson DC, Gilbert ES, Dores GM, et al. Long-term solid cancer risk among 5-year survivors of Hodgkin's lymphoma. J Clin Oncol 2007;25:1489–97.

[22] Travis LB, Hill DA, Dores GM, et al. Breast cancer following radiotherapy and chemotherapy among young women with Hodgkin disease. JAMA 2003;290:465–75.

[23] van Leeuwen FE, Klokman WJ, Stovall M, et al. Roles of radiation dose, chemotherapy, and hormonal factors in breast cancer following Hodgkin's disease. J Natl Cancer Inst 2003;95:971–80.

[24] Travis LB, Gospodarowicz M, Curtis RE, et al. Lung cancer following chemotherapy and radiotherapy for Hodgkin's disease. J Natl Cancer Inst 2002;94:182–92.

[25] Girinsky T, van der Maazen R, Specht L, et al. Involved-node radiotherapy (INRT) in patients with early Hodgkin lymphoma: concepts and guidelines. Radiother Oncol 2006;79:270–7.

[26] Swerdlow AJ, Barber JA, Hudson GV, et al. Risk of second malignancy after Hodgkin's disease in a collaborative British cohort: the relation to age at treatment. J Clin Oncol 2000;18:498–509.

[27] Swerdlow AJ, Schoemaker MJ, Allerton R, et al. Lung cancer after Hodgkin's disease: a nested case-control study of the relation to treatment. J Clin Oncol 2001;19:1610–8.

[28] van Leeuwen FE, Klokman WJ, Veer MB, et al. Long-term risk of second malignancy in survivors of Hodgkin's disease treated during adolescence or young adulthood. J Clin Oncol 2000;18:487–97.

[29] Aisenberg AC, Finkelstein DM, Doppke KP, et al. High risk of breast carcinoma after irradiation of young women with Hodgkin's disease. Cancer 1997;79:1203–10.

[30] Sankila R, Garwicz S, Olsen JH, et al. Risk of subsequent malignant neoplasms among 1,641 Hodgkin's disease patients diagnosed in childhood and adolescence: a population-based cohort study in the five Nordic countries. Association of the Nordic Cancer

Registries and the Nordic Society of Pediatric Hematology and Oncology. J Clin Oncol 1996;14:1442–6.

[31] Bhatia S, Yasui Y, Robison LL, et al. High risk of subsequent neoplasms continues with extended follow-up of childhood Hodgkin's disease: report from the Late Effects Study Group. J Clin Oncol 2003;21:4386–94.

[32] Gooley TA, Leisenring W, Crowley J, et al. Estimation of failure probabilities in the presence of competing risks: new representations of old estimators. Stat Med 1999;18:695–706.

[33] Gail MH, Brinton LA, Byar DP, et al. Projecting individualized probabilities of developing breast cancer for white females who are being examined annually. J Natl Cancer Inst 1989;81:1879–86.

[34] Travis LB, Hill D, Dores GM, et al. Cumulative absolute breast cancer risk for young women treated for Hodgkin lymphoma. J Natl Cancer Inst 2005;97:1428–37.

[35] Mauch P, Ng A, Aleman B, et al. Report from the Rockefeller Foundation sponsored international workshop on reducing mortality and improving quality of life in long-term survivors of Hodgkin's disease: July 9–16, 2003, Bellagio, Italy. Eur J Haematol 2005;75(Suppl):68–76.

[36] Andre M, Mounier N, Leleu X, et al. Second cancers and late toxicities after treatment of aggressive non-Hodgkin lymphoma with the ACVBP regimen: a GELA cohort study on 2837 patients. Blood 2004;103:1222–8.

[37] Mudie NY, Swerdlow AJ, Higgins CD, et al. Risk of second malignancy after non-Hodgkin's lymphoma: a British Cohort Study. J Clin Oncol 2006;24:1568–74.

[38] Tward JD, Wendland MM, Shrieve DC, et al. The risk of secondary malignancies over 30 years after the treatment of non-Hodgkin lymphoma. Cancer 2006;107:108–15.

[39] Freedman D, Curtis R, Travis L, et al. New malignancies following cancer of the uterine corpus and ovary. In: Curtis R, Freedman D, Ron E, et al, editors. New malignancies among cancer survivors: SEER cancer registries, 1973–2000 (NIH Publ. No. 05-5302). Bethesda (MD): National Institutes of Health; 2006. p. 231–55.

[40] Curtis RE, Metayer C, Rizzo JD, et al. Impact of chronic GVHD therapy on the development of squamous-cell cancers after hematopoietic stem-cell transplantation: an international case-control study. Blood 2005;105:3802–11.

[41] Travis LB, Curtis RE, Boice JD Jr, et al. Second cancers following non-Hodgkin's lymphoma. Cancer 1991;67:2002–9.

[42] Travis LB, Gonzalez CL, Hankey BF, et al. Hodgkin's disease following non-Hodgkin's lymphoma. Cancer 1992;69:2337–42.

[43] Travis LB, Holowaty E, Hunter V, et al. Acute basophilic leukemia and acute eosinophilic leukemia after therapy for non-Hodgkin's lymphoma. Am J Clin Pathol 1993;100:186.

[44] Travis LB, Curtis RE, Glimelius B, et al. Second cancers among long-term survivors of non-Hodgkin's lymphoma. J Natl Cancer Inst 1993;85:1932–7.

[45] Travis LB, Curtis RE, Glimelius B, et al. Bladder and kidney cancer following cyclophospha-mide therapy for non-Hodgkin's lymphoma. J Natl Cancer Inst 1995;87:524–30.

[46] Bonnet C, Fillet G, Mounier N, et al. CHOP alone compared with CHOP plus radiotherapy for localized aggressive lymphoma in elderly patients: a study by the Groupe d'Etude des Lymphomes de l'Adulte. J Clin Oncol 2007;25:787–92.

[47] Shenkier TN, Voss N, Fairey R, et al. Brief chemotherapy and involved-region irradiation for limited-stage diffuse large-cell lymphoma: an 18-year experience from the British Columbia Cancer Agency. J Clin Oncol 2002;20:197–204.

[48] Schairer C, Hisada M, Chen BE, et al. Comparative mortality for 621 second cancers in 29,356 testicular cancer survivors and 12,420 matched first cancers. J Natl Cancer Inst 2007;99:1248–56.

[49] van den Belt-Dusebout AW, de Wit R, Gietema JA, et al. Treatment-specific risks of second malignancies and cardiovascular disease in 5-year survivors of testicular cancer. J Clin Oncol 2007;25:4370–8.

[50] Travis LB, Fossa SD, Schonfeld SJ, et al. Second cancers among 40,576 testicular cancer patients: focus on long-term survivors. J Natl Cancer Inst 2005;97:1354–65.

[51] Fossa SD, Chen J, Schonfeld SJ, et al. Risk of contralateral testicular cancer: a population-based study of 29,515 U.S. men. J Natl Cancer Inst 2005;97:1056–66.

[52] Travis LB, Andersson M, Gospodarowicz M, et al. Treatment-associated leukemia following testicular cancer. J Natl Cancer Inst 2000;92:1165–71.

[53] Pedersen-Bjergaard J, Daugaard G, Hansen SW, et al. Increased risk of myelodysplasia and leukemia after etoposide, cisplatin, and bleomycin for germ-cell tumours. Lancet 1991;338:359–63.

[54] Kollmannsberger C, Hartmann JT, Kanz L, et al. Therapy-related malignancies following treatment of germ cell cancer. Int J Cancer 1999;83:860–3.

[55] Kirova YM, Gambotti L, De Rycke Y, et al. Risk of second malignancies after adjuvant radiotherapy for breast cancer: a large-scale, single-institution review. Int J Radiat Oncol Biol Phys 2007;68:359–63.

[56] Gao X, Fisher SG, Emami B. Risk of second primary cancer in the contralateral breast in women treated for early-stage breast cancer: a population-based study. Int J Radiat Oncol Biol Phys 2003;56:1038–45.

[57] Hemminki K, Ji J, Forsti A. Risks for familial and contralateral breast cancer interact multiplicatively and cause a high risk. Cancer Res 2007;67:868–70.

[58] Boice JD Jr, Harvey EB, Blettner M, et al. Cancer in the contralateral breast after radiotherapy for breast cancer. N Engl J Med 1992;326:781–5.

[59] Storm HH, Andersson M, Boice JD Jr, et al. Adjuvant radiotherapy and risk of contralateral breast cancer. J Natl Cancer Inst 1992;84:1245–50.

[60] Hill-Kayser CE, Harris EE, Hwang WT, et al. Twenty-year incidence and patterns of contralateral breast cancer after breast conservation treatment with radiation. Int J Radiat Oncol Biol Phys 2006;66:1313–9.

[61] Clarke M, Collins R, Darby S, et al. Effects of radiotherapy and of differences in the extent of surgery for early breast cancer on local recurrence and 15-year survival: an overview of the randomised trials. Lancet 2005;366:2087–106.

[62] Early Breast Cancer Trialists' Collaborative Group (EBDTCG). Effects of chemotherapy and hormonal therapy for early breast cancer on recurrence and 15-year survival: an overview of the randomised trials. Lancet 2005;365:1687–717.

[63] Fisher B, Costantino JP, Redmond CK, et al. Endometrial cancer in tamoxifen-treated breast cancer patients: findings from the National Surgical Adjuvant Breast and Bowel Project (NSABP) B-14 [see comments]. J Natl Cancer Inst 1994;86:527–37.

[64] Fisher B, Costantino JP, Wickerham DL, et al. Tamoxifen for prevention of breast cancer: report of the National Surgical Adjuvant Breast and Bowel Project P-1 Study [see comments]. J Natl Cancer Inst 1998;90:1371–88.

[65] Magriples U, Naftolin F, Schwartz PE, et al. High-grade endometrial carcinoma in tamoxifen-treated breast cancer patients. J Clin Oncol 1993;11:485–90.

[66] Bergman L, Beelen ML, Gallee MP, et al. Risk and prognosis of endometrial cancer after tamoxifen for breast cancer. Comprehensive Cancer Centres' ALERT Group. Assessment of liver and endometrial cancer risk following tamoxifen. Lancet 2000;356:881–7.

[67] Saadat M, Truong PT, Kader HA, et al. Outcomes in patients with primary breast cancer and a subsequent diagnosis of endometrial cancer: comparison of cohorts treated with and without tamoxifen. Cancer 2007;110:31–7.

[68] Roychoudhuri R, Evans H, Robinson D, et al. Radiation-induced malignancies following radiotherapy for breast cancer. Br J Cancer 2004;91:868–72.

[69] Neugut AI, Robinson E, Lee WC, et al. Lung cancer after radiation therapy for breast cancer [see comments]. Cancer 1993;71:3054–7.

[70] Zablotska LB, Neugut AI. Lung carcinoma after radiation therapy in women treated with lumpectomy or mastectomy for primary breast carcinoma. Cancer 2003;97:1404–11.

[71] Deutsch M, Land SR, Begovic M, et al. The incidence of lung carcinoma after surgery for breast carcinoma with and without postoperative radiotherapy. Results of National Surgical Adjuvant Breast and Bowel Project (NSABP) clinical trials B-04 and B-06. Cancer 2003;98:1362–8.

[72] Neugut AI, Murray T, Santos J, et al. Increased risk of lung cancer after breast cancer radiation therapy in cigarette smokers [see comments]. Cancer 1994;73:1615–20.

[73] Ford MB, Sigurdson AJ, Petrulis ES, et al. Effects of smoking and radiotherapy on lung carcinoma in breast carcinoma survivors. Cancer 2003;98:1457–64.

[74] Huang J, Mackillop WJ. Increased risk of soft tissue sarcoma after radiotherapy in women with breast carcinoma. Cancer 2001;92:172–80.

[75] Karlsson P, Holmberg E, Samuelsson A, et al. Soft tissue sarcoma after treatment for breast cancer—a Swedish population-based study. Eur J Cancer 1998;34:2068–75.

[76] Kirova YM, Vilcoq JR, Asselain B, et al. Radiation-induced sarcomas after radiotherapy for breast carcinoma: a large-scale single-institution review. Cancer 2005;104:856–63.

[77] Rubino C, de Vathaire F, Shamsaldin A, et al. Radiation dose, chemotherapy, hormonal treatment and risk of second cancer after breast cancer treatment. Br J Cancer 2003;89:840–6.

[78] Jessner M, Zak FG, Rein CR. Angiosarcoma in postmastectomy lymphedema (Stewart-Treves syndrome). AMA Arch Derm Syphilol 1952;65:123–9.

[79] Esler-Brauer L, Jaggernauth W, Zeitouni NC. Angiosarcoma developing after conservative treatment for breast carcinoma: case report with review of the current literature. Dermatol Surg 2007;33:749–55.

[80] Virtanen A, Pukkala E, Auvinen A. Angiosarcoma after radiotherapy: a cohort study of 332,163 Finnish cancer patients. Br J Cancer 2007;97:115–7.

[81] Simonart T, Heenen M. Radiation-induced angiosarcomas. Dermatology 2004;209:175–6.

[82] Curtis RE, Boice JD Jr, Stovall M, et al. Risk of leukemia after chemotherapy and radiation treatment for breast cancer. N Engl J Med 1992;326:1745–51.

[83] Praga C, Bergh J, Bliss J, et al. Risk of acute myeloid leukemia and myelodysplastic syndrome in trials of adjuvant epirubicin for early breast cancer: correlation with doses of epirubicin and cyclophosphamide. J Clin Oncol 2005;23:4179–91.

[84] Campone M, Roche H, Kerbrat P, et al. Secondary leukemia after epirubicin-based adjuvant chemotherapy in operable breast cancer patients: 16 years experience of the French Adjuvant Study Group. Ann Oncol 2005;16:1343–51.

[85] Park MJ, Park YH, Ahn HJ, et al. Secondary hematological malignancies after breast cancer chemotherapy. Leuk Lymphoma 2005;46:1183–8.

[86] Smith RE, Bryant J, DeCillis A, et al. Acute myeloid leukemia and myelodysplastic syndrome after doxorubicin-cyclophosphamide adjuvant therapy for operable breast cancer: the National Surgical Adjuvant Breast and Bowel Project Experience. J Clin Oncol 2003;21:1195–204.

[87] Chen PY, Vicini FA. Partial breast irradiation. Patient selection, guidelines for treatment, and current results. Front Radiat Ther Oncol 2007;40:253–71.

[88] Liauw SL, Sylvester JE, Morris CG, et al. Second malignancies after prostate brachytherapy: incidence of bladder and colorectal cancers in patients with 15 years of potential follow-up. Int J Radiat Oncol Biol Phys 2006;66:669–73.

[89] Moon K, Stukenborg GJ, Keim J, et al. Cancer incidence after localized therapy for prostate cancer. Cancer 2006;107:991–8.

[90] Kendal WS, Eapen L, Macrae R, et al. Prostatic irradiation is not associated with any measurable increase in the risk of subsequent rectal cancer. Int J Radiat Oncol Biol Phys 2006;65:661–8.

[91] Chrouser K, Leibovich B, Bergstralh E, et al. Bladder cancer risk following primary and adjuvant external beam radiation for prostate cancer. J Urol 2005;174:107–10 [discussion: 110–11].

[92] Hall EJ, Wuu CS. Radiation-induced second cancers: the impact of 3D-CRT and IMRT. Int J Radiat Oncol Biol Phys 2003;56:83–8.

[93] Pickles T, Phillips N. The risk of second malignancy in men with prostate cancer treated with or without radiation in British Columbia, 1984–2000. Radiother Oncol 2002;65: 145–51.

[94] Brenner DJ, Curtis RE, Hall EJ, et al. Second malignancies in prostate carcinoma patients after radiotherapy compared with surgery. Cancer 2000;88:398–406.

[95] Neugut AI, Ahsan H, Robinson E, et al. Bladder carcinoma and other second malignancies after radiotherapy for prostate carcinoma. Cancer 1997;79:1600–4.

[96] Guckenberger M, Flentje M. Intensity-modulated radiotherapy (IMRT) of localized prostate cancer: a review and future perspectives. Strahlenther Onkol 2007;183:57–62.

[97] Kry SF, Salehpour M, Followill DS, et al. The calculated risk of fatal secondary malignancies from intensity-modulated radiation therapy. Int J Radiat Oncol Biol Phys 2005;62: 1195–203.

[98] Kleinerman RA, Curtis RE, Boice JD Jr, et al. Second cancers following radiotherapy for cervical cancer. J Natl Cancer Inst 1982;69:1027–33.

[99] Kleinerman RA, Boice JD Jr, Storm HH, et al. Second primary cancer after treatment for cervical cancer. An international cancer registries study. Cancer 1995;76:442–52.

[100] Boice JD Jr, Engholm G, Kleinerman RA, et al. Radiation dose and second cancer risk in patients treated for cancer of the cervix. Radiat Res 1988;116:3–55.

[101] Boice JD Jr, Blettner M, Kleinerman RA, et al. Radiation dose and leukemia risk in patients treated for cancer of the cervix. J Natl Cancer Inst 1987;79:1295–311.

[102] Chaturvedi AK, Engels EA, Gilbert ES, et al. Second cancers among 104,760 survivors of cervical cancer: evaluation of long-term risk. J Natl Cancer Inst 2007;99:1634–43.

[103] Keys HM, Bundy BN, Stehman FB, et al. Cisplatin, radiation, and adjuvant hysterectomy compared with radiation and adjuvant hysterectomy for bulky stage IB cervical carcinoma. N Engl J Med 1999;340:1154–61.

[104] Rose PG, Bundy BN, Watkins EB, et al. Concurrent cisplatin-based radiotherapy and chemotherapy for locally advanced cervical cancer. N Engl J Med 1999;340: 1144–53.

[105] Morris M, Eifel PJ, Lu J, et al. Pelvic radiation with concurrent chemotherapy compared with pelvic and para-aortic radiation for high-risk cervical cancer. N Engl J Med 1999;340: 1137–43.

[106] Poirier MC, Reed E, Litterst CL, et al. Persistence of platinum-ammine-DNA adducts in gonads and kidneys of rats and multiple tissues from cancer patients. Cancer Res 1992;52:149–53.

[107] Greene MH. Is cisplatin a human carcinogen? J Natl Cancer Inst 1992;84:306–12.

[108] Travis LB, Holowaty EJ, Bergfeldt K, et al. Risk of leukemia after platinum-based chemotherapy for ovarian cancer. N Engl J Med 1999;340:351–7.

[109] Leon X, Ferlito A, Myer CM 3rd, et al. Second primary tumors in head and neck cancer patients. Acta Otolaryngol 2002;122:765–78.

[110] Gallo O, Sardi I, Pepe G, et al. Multiple primary tumors of the upper aerodigestive tract: is there a role for constitutional mutations in the p53 gene? Int J Cancer 1999;82: 180–6.

[111] Cianfriglia F, Di Gregorio DA, Manieri A. Multiple primary tumours in patients with oral squamous cell carcinoma. Oral Oncol 1999;35:157–63.

[112] Leon X, Quer M, Diez S, et al. Second neoplasm in patients with head and neck cancer. Head Neck 1999;21:204–10.

[113] Rinaldo A, Marchiori C, Faggionato L, et al. The association of cancers of the larynx with cancers of the lung. Eur Arch Otorhinolaryngol 1996;253:256–9.

[114] Berg JW, Schottenfeld D, Ritter F. Incidence of multiple primary cancers. III. Cancers of the respiratory and upper digestive system as multiple primary cancers. J Natl Cancer Inst 1970;44:263–74.

[115] Day GL, Blot WJ, Shore RE, et al. Second cancers following oral and pharyngeal cancers: role of tobacco and alcohol. J Natl Cancer Inst 1994;86:131–7.
[116] Bongers V, Braakhuis BJ, Tobi H, et al. The relation between cancer incidence among relatives and the occurrence of multiple primary carcinomas following head and neck cancer. Cancer Epidemiol Biomarkers Prev 1996;5:595–8.
[117] Jain S, Khuri FR, Shin DM. Prevention of head and neck cancer: current status and future prospects. Curr Probl Cancer 2004;28:265–86.
[118] Smith W, Saba N. Retinoids as chemoprevention for head and neck cancer: where do we go from here? Crit Rev Oncol Hematol 2005;55:143–52.

Fertility and Sexuality in Young Cancer Survivors Who Have Adult-Onset Malignancies

Sophie D. Fosså, MD, PhD[a,b,*], Alv A. Dahl, MD, PhD[a,b]

[a]Department of Clinical Cancer Research, The Norwegian Radium Hospital, Rikshospitalet University Hospital, Montebello, 0310 Oslo, Norway
[b]Faculty Division, The Norwegian Radium Hospital, University of Oslo, 0316 Oslo, Norway

Approximately 7% of malignant tumors are diagnosed in individuals aged 15 to 44 years old (males: 5%; females: 9% of adult-onset malignancies). The most frequent diagnoses in males are testicular cancer (TC) and Hodgkin lymphoma (HL), and in females, breast and cervical cancer [1]. Most cases require multimodal therapy. In these young patients clinicians have to consider how the planned treatment affects the patient's probability of future parenthood, particularly in light of the recent tendency to delay family building to the fourth decade of life or even later. Even patients who have completed their families are concerned with the possible influence of cancer treatment on their future sexual lives. This article provides a summary of current knowledge about posttreatment reproduction and sexuality mainly concerning tumor-free cancer survivors diagnosed with cancer between the ages of 15 and 44 years.

PHYSIOLOGY
Males
The endocrine and exocrine testicular function depends on regulation by the pituitary gonadotropins: LH (for testosterone) and FSH (for spermatogenesis). Secondary hypogonadism develops after high-dose cranial radiotherapy because of abolished production of these gonadotropins. Orchiectomy, testicular radiotherapy, or selected cytostatics may lead to primary hypogonadism as a result of reduced number of spermatogonia or Leydig cells. The gonadotoxic effect depends on the type of chemotherapy, cumulative doses, or testicular radiation doses. Recovery of spermatogenesis can be expected as long as some spermatogonia are preserved. Testicular radiation of 4 to 6 Gy is followed by permanent azoospermia. An undisturbed transport of mature sperm

*Corresponding author. Department of Clinical Cancer Research, The Norwegian Radium Hospital, Rikshospitalet University Hospital, Montebello, 0310 Oslo, Norway. E-mail address: sdf@radiumhospitalet.no (S.D. Fosså).

0889-8588/08/$ – see front matter
doi:10.1016/j.hoc.2008.01.002
hemonc.theclinics.com

cells mediated by erection and ejaculation is required for the "natural" initiation of a pregnancy.

Females

Estrogen and progesterone are produced by the maturing primordial follicle during the menstrual cycle. The number of primordial follicles in the ovaries is defined during embryonal life and decreases gradually with postnatal aging. A normal pituitary function is mandatory for an ovulatory menstrual cycle. High-dose cranial radiotherapy thus could lead to secondary ovarian failure. Cytotoxic therapy leads to an increased removal of primordial follicles, which are not able to renew themselves. The type and dose of cytostatic drugs or radiation and age predict the risk for premature ovarian failure (POF) (permanent ovarian failure before the age of 41 years is estimated to occur following ovarian radiation at a dose of 14 Gy given at age 30 [2]). Further, physiologic pregnancy requires undisturbed transport of the mature ovum and nidation together with a normal uterine anatomy and function, processes that may be disturbed by pelvic surgery or radiation.

FERTILITY IN YOUNG CANCER SURVIVORS

General

Compared with the general population cancer survivors' postdiagnosis reproduction may be reduced by medical reasons that decrease the possibility to initiate and go through a pregnancy or psychosocial reasons leading to reduced desire and attempts to initiate a pregnancy [3].

Recent medical literature contains multiple reports on postcancer reproduction mirrored by recovery of sperm counts or serum FSH, and achieved pregnancies of cancer, for example after HL [4–10], TC [11,12], cervical cancer [13,14], or breast cancer [15]. These studies show that 60% to 70% of survivors of HL and TC who attempt posttreatment parenthood are successful without assisted reproduction techniques. The 10-year first-time postdiagnosis reproduction rate in males who are childless at the time of the malignant diagnosis is significantly higher than that of the general population (Table 1) [16]. Pregnancies in female cancer survivors display a significantly higher risk for preterm delivery and low birth weight [13,17]. Whether there is an increased risk for congenital abnormalities in the offspring of cancer survivors is still a matter of ongoing debate [17,18]. Female cancer survivors' postdiagnosis reproduction rates were, however, significantly less than those of the general population [17]. Finally, there is no risk that cancer-specific mortality increases because of pregnancies after the malignant diagnosis [15,19].

Specific Diagnoses

Testicular cancer

Approximately two thirds of patients who have newly diagnosed TC do not exclude future fatherhood [20], which in approximately 20% of the patients is threatened by the pre-existing hypogonadism related to the testicular dysgenesis syndrome [21]. Necessary anticancer therapy may further reduce the

Table 1
Cumulative relative probability and hazards ratios of first postdiagnosis reproduction in individuals aged 15 to 44 years at their cancer diagnosis (1971–1997)

	All		Malignant lymphoma/leukemia		Testicular cancer	Gynecologic cancer	Breast cancer
	Males 2722	Females 3349	Males 618	Females 415	1139	1468	638
No. of patients							
All 10-CRP	0.32/0.28ᵃ	0.12/0.22	0.35/0.29ᵃ	0.28/0.35	0.34/0.31ᵃ	0.06/0.21	0.05/0.10
HR (95% CI)	1.2 (1.10–1.30)ᵃ	0.52 (0.47–0.58)	1.24 (1.05–1.46)ᵃ	0.8 (0.65–0.98)	1.12 (1.0–1.26)ᵃ	0.26 (0.21–0.31)	0.50 (0.36–0.69)
Childless 10-CRP	0.34/0.24ᵃ	0.25/0.30	0.37/0.28ᵃ	0.42/0.40	0.35/0.25ᵃ	0.13/0.27	0.12/0.11
One prior child 10-CRP	0.46/0.63	0.14/0.39	0.42/0.68	0.34/0.59	0.50/0.66	0.08/0.40	0.06/0.20
Two or more prior children 10-CRP	0.13/0.21	0.02/0.09	0.15/0.2	0.02/0.12	0.14/0.28	0.01/0.11	0.02/0.05

HRs are adjusted for age of diagnosis and extent of the disease. CRPs are expressed as cancer patients/controls.

Abbreviations: 10-CRP, 10-year cumulative relative probability; HR, hazard ratio.

ᵃP ≤ .05.

Data from Cvancarova MS, Magelssen H, Fosså SD. Ten-year reproduction rates (10-RR) after cancer treatment: comparison between patients (cases) and the normal population (controls). J Clin Oncol 2007;25(185):9075.

chance of postcancer paternity. Approximately 2 years after modern cisplatin-based standard chemotherapy, however, spermatogenesis has recovered in at least 80% of testicular cancer survivors (TCSs) with sperm counts sufficient for initiation of a pregnancy [11]. These observed sperm counts are comparable to the 80% 15-year paternity rate in TCSs who have antegrade ejaculation who successfully attempt posttreatment fatherhood [12].

Modern fertility-saving treatment of TC (appropriate testicular shielding during radiotherapy [22], reduced radiation doses and target fields [23], wait-and-see policy [24], nerve-sparing operations [25]) have been followed by improved postdiagnosis reproduction rates after 1990 (Fig. 1A).

Hodgkin lymphoma
The mean age of males who have HL at the time diagnosis is 30 years, and about 50% of the patients have at least one child before the start of anticancer treatment [10]. Previously, MOPP (mustargen, oncovin, procarbazine, and prednisone) therapy was followed by permanent infertility in more than 90% of male Hodgkin lymphoma survivors (HLSs) [10]. After introduction of the ABVD (adriamycin, bleomycin, vinblastine, DTIC) treatment and omission of alkylating agent–based therapies, approximately 80% of elevated FSH values become normal in HLSs, indicating a recovery of spermatogenesis [8]. This experience is mirrored by an approximately 60% 10-year cumulative rate of fatherhood in HLSs who attempted posttreatment paternity [9].

The introduction of ABVD chemotherapy and avoidance of pelvic radiotherapy have increased the chances of physiologic posttreatment motherhood in approximately 80% of female HLSs who attempted pregnancy [9]. Even women who regain menstrual cycles after treatment are at risk for developing POF after 15 to 20 years of observation, however [26]. The highest risk for POF is for patients diagnosed after the age of 30 years.

Breast cancer
Approximately 10% of breast cancer diagnoses are made in women younger than 45 years of age. For most of them, the question of future postdiagnosis motherhood is not relevant because they have completed their families. Many women now delay motherhood to an age of 30 to 35 years, however. Because of adjuvant cytostatic treatment and several years of hormone therapy the 10-year cumulative rate of postdiagnosis pregnancies is low (see Table 1), although childbirth has been reported after CMF (cyclophosphamide, methotrexate, 5-fluoro-uracil) and FEC (5-fluoro-uracil, epirubicin, cyclophosphamide) treatments, even when combined with tamoxifen. Several studies have shown that postdiagnosis pregnancies do not affect cancer-specific survival [15,19].

Gynecologic cancer
Approximately 40% of women who have cervical cancer and 9% of those who have ovarian cancer are younger than 45 years of age. Because their treatment often consists of resections of the reproductive organs or high-dose pelvic radiotherapy posttreatment reproduction rates are very low (see Table 1). Some

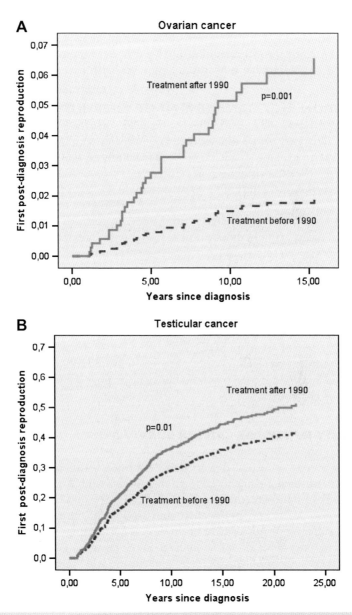

Fig. 1. Cumulative probability for first postdiagnosis reproduction in patients who have cancer diagnosed from age 15 to 44 years, and during 1971 to 1990 compared with 1991 to 1997. (A) Ovarian cancer. (B) Testicular cancer.

improvement has been observed after the introduction of fertility-saving surgery (Fig. 1B) [13,14]. Cisplatin-based chemotherapy of ovarian germ cell cancer [27] and treatment with methotrexate for choriocarcinoma [28] is followed by recovery of the ovarian function in almost all patients.

PREVENTION AND MANAGEMENT OF INFERTILITY

In all patients who have a new malignant diagnosis the risk for future infertility should be discussed before treatment starts. In males who have a new cancer diagnosis sperm banking should be encouraged. Only 15% to 20% of male cancer survivors ever use their deep-frozen semen, however [20]. If pelvic radiotherapy becomes necessary the testicles should be shielded appropriately [22]. Whenever possible, orchiectomy because of bilateral TC surgery should consist of a unilateral organ-saving resection [29]. Assisted fertilization may lead to postdiagnosis fatherhood in males persistently infertile after treatment using cryopreserved semen, ejaculated oligospermic semen, or semen extracted from the testicles [30].

Fewer and less effective preventive tasks are available for women [31]. The effect of oophoropexy before pelvic irradiation is reduced by subsequent migration of the ovaries or disturbances of their blood circulation. Ovarian autotransplantation can protect against radiation-induced ovarian failure [31]. Pretreatment cryopreservation of ovarian tissue is today increasingly offered [31], with a few successful pregnancies reported. There is some indication for a protective effect of luteinizing hormone releasing hormone analogs applied together with gonadotoxic chemotherapy [32].

SEXUALITY IN YOUNG CANCER SURVIVORS
General

The many studies of sexual dysfunction performed between 1990 and 2000 clearly demonstrated the methodologic pitfalls in this field [33]. Common problems are lack of standard criteria for sexual dysfunction and lack of separation of dysfunction per se and dysfunction with significant consequences, such as subjective suffering or impairment of the sexual partnership. Further, it is still undecided if interviews or questionnaires give the most valid information. These methodologic problems partially explain the wide interstudy variation in prevalence rates for sexual dysfunctions.

Two conclusions seem valid from the prevalence studies: (1) Sexual dysfunctions are common in the general population, and (2) they regularly increase with age [33,34]. Further, sexuality is influenced by medical, physiologic, emotional, relationship, and social expectancy factors, many of which are affected by cancer illness experiences, such as treatment, fear of relapse, and risk for infertility. In the increasingly multicultural societies of Europe and the United States it is also important to consider minorities' religious, cultural, and sexual traditions when sexual matters are considered [35].

Compared with the general population cancer survivors' postdiagnosis motivation and ability for sexual activity may be affected by:

Medical reasons that decrease former pleasure and satisfaction. Medication used to treat depression, anxiety, pain, and nausea often have sexual side effects.

Psychosocial reasons caused by changes in the sexual organs, body image, and sex roles, and the sexual responses of the partner.

Major treatment sequelae that may reduce the chances of finding a sexual partner.

High threshold for seeking help in such intimate and sensitive matters. Physicians and nurses are generally reluctant to bring up issues related to sexuality, and they do not create an atmosphere that invites the patients to bring up such matters [36].

Male Sexuality

In males a physiologic model of arousal, plateau, orgasm, and resolution still is considered valid. In contrast, physiologic reactions are considered less important than contextual and intimate factors for the sexual response cycle in females [37].

Specific diagnoses

Testicular cancer. In most studies 70% to 90% of TCSs were in partnered relationships when TC was diagnosed. The rate of divorce and broken relationships is 5% to 10% in most follow-up studies, and these couples saw the cancer as a significant factor in their break-up [38]. The main concern of the wives was to become pregnant, particularly if the couple did not have children before the TC was diagnosed.

In their review of 36 studies of sexuality in TCSs, Jonker-Pool and colleagues [39] concluded: "It is very difficult to make a clear picture based on the outcome of the existing studies," and Nazareth and colleagues [40] stated that: "Better evidence is needed in studies that control for the impact of the testicular cancer, the treatment modality and psychologic reactions to both." Overall Jonker-Pool and colleagues found that 20% of TCSs had lack of desire, 12% had erectile disorder, 44% ejaculation disorder, and 19% sexual dissatisfaction. Except for ejaculation disorder, these prevalence rates hardly differed from normative American data [41]. The review concluded that reduced function in the psychologic domains (drive, satisfaction) was treatment independent, whereas changes in physiologic domains (erection, ejaculation) were associated with extent of disease and treatment modalities. Based on six controlled studies, Nazareth and colleagues [40] calculated that the odds ratios for TCSs compared with controls were 1.6 (95% CI 1.1–2.3) for lack of drive, 2.6 (95% CI 1.6–4.1) for erectile dysfunction, and 13.7 (95% CI 7.9–23.9) for ejaculatory dysfunction.

Generally, there seems to be a high correlation between sexual functioning before and after treatment of TC [42,43]. Findings must be considered in relation to age [44] and to the prevalence in the general population.

A national multicenter study from Norway [45] confirmed the findings showing significantly worse scores on ejaculatory function in TCSs compared with the general population. In this study overall sexual problems were observed in 35% of the young TCSs (20–39 years; norm: 29%) and among 41% of the middle-aged group (40–59 years; norm: 40%). In multivariate analyses, overall sexual problems in TCSs were significantly associated with increasing age, being without partner, and a higher anxiety score, whereas ejaculation problems showed significant association with no partner and a trend for chemotherapy and neurotoxic side effects. The findings of Jonker-Pool and colleagues [39] that the psychologic domains of drive and satisfaction were treatment-independent were also confirmed, but in contrast to these authors the physiologic function of erection was found to have no relation to treatment.

Hodgkin lymphoma. In the few studies on sexuality among survivors after HL approximately 20% of the patients [46–48] complained of sexual problems. There is reason to believe that fatigue and somatic symptoms after chemotherapy influence sexuality, and the same is relevant for the emotional distress and partner reactions associated with diagnosis and treatment of the disease. The fertility issue may also eventually affect the sexual life of the couple.

Female Sexuality

Recently Basson [49] conceptualized the female sexual response as a cyclical reinforcement model in which intimacy and emotional factors were more important than for male sexuality. Women may thus instigate physical contact or be receptive to sexual initiation for various reasons, such as desire for closeness, intimacy, commitment, or as an expression of caring. Basson thus emphasized the stronger influence of psychologic and contextual factors in females rather than the biologic ones (experience of orgasm and resolution). This complexity of female sexuality is expressed in the multiple etiologic factors and determinants of sexual problems and has to be taken into account when sexuality after cancer is considered in females.

Specific diagnoses
Breast cancer. Although there is a considerable literature on the sexuality of patients who have breast cancer in general, there are few studies that specifically examine younger (≤50 years) patients. Breast cancer did not seem to imply an increased rate of marital breakdowns [50]. The cancer experience frequently strengthened the relationship [51]. The sexual interest of the partner and the quality of first sexual experiences after treatment were also important [52]. Many men have problems addressing distressing interpersonal issues with their female partners, however, and thus they avoid communications about sexuality [53].

No significant differences have been observed as to the associations between sexual problems and lumpectomy or mastectomy [54]. Chemotherapy can lead to premature menopause, and hormonal treatment can worsen menopausal symptoms. Time since treatment also is an important factor as is the age of the patient. Finally, the sexual functioning before onset of cancer is of relevance.

Burwell and colleagues [55] in a prospective study of young breast cancer survivors found that the sexual problems at 1 year post-surgery were significantly higher than before diagnosis. In multivariable analyses controlling for sexual problems at prediagnosis, vaginal dryness and lower perceived sexual attractiveness were consistently associated with greater overall sexual problems. Chemotherapy was related to sexual problems only early after surgery except for women who became menopausal as a result of chemotherapy and who continued to have problems.

In another study of younger patients, Fobair and colleagues [56] found that 67% were sexually active during the first year after treatment. Among them about 33% reported having no sexual problems, 15% had few problems, and 52% reported more definite or serious problems. The most common reason for being sexually inactive was lack of interest (50%), physical problems, or being too tired. The proportion of sexually active women in the study of the younger patients was comparable to the 65% of breast cancer survivors reporting sexual problems who participated in a study that included all age groups [57].

In comparing young women who had breast cancer with women of similar age who did not have breast cancer, cancer patients showed significantly reduced sexual activity and higher prevalence of problems, such as lack of arousal and inability to enjoy sex, vaginal dryness, and hot flashes. Poor mental health and impaired quality of the relationship with the partner were also associated with sexual problems [58]. These problems remained even during long-term follow-up [57,59]. Younger women who had been cancer-free for 5 years still did not show improvement in sexual activity or problems [54].

Among young women sexual problems, marital problems, and concerns about body image were predictive of overall quality of life [60]. The findings concerning younger women underscore the importance of counseling them and their partners about the expected consequences of treatment-related side effects on their intimate relationship. The partner's view and behavior are of major relevance for feelings of sexual attractiveness in the female.

Cervical cancer. There are few studies that also involve the partners of women who have cervical cancer. In a small study, De Groot and colleagues [61] found that male partners expressed a strong wish to be involved in and informed about the illness of their spouses.

Overall sexual problems were significantly more common in women who had cancer compared with controls, although sexual partnership and activity did not differ [62]. Differences between studies are obvious, however. A study from Sweden showed that 68% of the patients treated for cervical cancer had regular intercourse 5 years after treatment, and that this prevalence did not differ from that of age-matched controls [62]. In contrast, studies from Denmark found a significantly reduced sexual interest in women who had cervical cancer compared with age-matched controls 2 years after treatment [63,64]. Communication with physicians about the sexual problems was associated with significantly reduced likelihood of sexual problems [65].

Women treated with radiation had significantly worse outcome on all sexual function parameters compared with women treated with surgery [66]. The latter women did not differ from cancer-free controls on any parameter [67]. After early stages of cervical cancer the quality of partnered relation, perceived physical appearance, and vaginal changes were significantly associated with sexual problems [68].

Ovarian cancer. To the knowledge of the authors, there are no studies of partners' reaction to ovarian cancer in their spouses, and no studies of couples. Three recent studies of sexuality in ovarian cancer survivors conclude that at least 2 years after primary treatment approximately half of the patients are sexually active [69–71]. This proportion does not differ significantly from age-matched controls who do not have cancer. The ovarian cancer survivors showed significantly less sexual pleasure and more discomfort compared with such controls, however [70,71]. Lack of interest and physical problems were significantly more common in sexually inactive patients compared with controls. In multivariable analyses being sexually inactive was significantly associated with premenopausal surgery, chemotherapy, age, mental health, and body image [71].

PREVENTION AND MANAGEMENT OF SEXUAL DYSFUNCTION

Several treatment-related issues are relevant for the sexual functioning in young cancer survivors. Nerve-sparing modifications of surgical techniques have reduced the prevalence of erectile and ejaculatory problems in testicular cancer survivors [25]. Because chemotherapy frequently is associated with increased prevalence of sexual problems, treatment should be based on risk-adapted strategies for maximal reduction of sexual problems with cure as the primary objective.

The major role of the partners' attitudes and approaches concerning the sexual functioning of the patients has been convincingly demonstrated in breast cancer. Corresponding data are not currently available for testicular or gynecologic cancer. There is no reason to believe, however, that the role of partner and relationship is less significant in these cancers, given its relevance for both male and female sexual response. Offers of counseling concerning sexual problems in relation to cancer treatment seem important along with a more open attitude toward sexual problems in oncologists and oncology nurses.

SUMMARY

For the clinical oncologist fertility and sexuality are important issues to consider together with the young patient who has cancer before treatment and during follow-up. There are today several options to enable post-cancer parenthood, particularly in males. Post-cancer sexuality may be improved both in males and females by inclusion of the partner in counseling.

References
[1] Cancer Registry of Norway: Cancer in Norway 2005. Available at: www. cancerregistry.no. Accessed December 21, 2006.
[2] Wallace WH, Thomson AB, Saran F, et al. Predicting age of ovarian failure after radiation to a field that includes the ovaries. Int J Radiat Oncol Biol Phys 2005;62:738–44.

[3] Schover LR. Psychosocial aspects of infertility and decisions about reproduction in young cancer survivors: a review. Med Pediatr Oncol 1999;33:53–9.

[4] Dubey P, Wilson G, Mathur KK, et al. Recovery of sperm production following radiation therapy for Hodgkin's disease after induction chemotherapy with mitoxantrone, vincristine, vinblastine, and prednisone (NOVP). Int J Radiat Oncol Biol Phys 2000;46:609–17.

[5] Franchi-Rezgui P, Rousselot P, Espié M, et al. Fertility in young women after chemotherapy with alkylating agents for Hodgkin and non-Hodgkin lymphomas. Hematol J 2003;4:116–20.

[6] Behringer K, Breuer K, Reineke T, et al. Secondary amenorrhea after Hodgkin's lymphoma is influenced by age at treatment, stage of disease, chemotherapy regimen, and the use of oral contraceptives during therapy: a report from the German Hodgkin's Lymphoma Study Group. J Clin Oncol 2005;23:7555–64.

[7] Hodgson DC, Pintilie M, Gitterman L, et al. Fertility among female Hodgkin lymphoma survivors attempting pregnancy following ABVD chemotherapy. Hematol Oncol 2007;25:11–5.

[8] van der Kaaij MA, Heutte N, Le Stang N, et al. Gonadal function in males after chemotherapy for early-stage Hodgkin's lymphoma treated in four subsequent trials by the European Organisation for Research and Treatment of Cancer: EORTC Lymphoma Group and the Groupe d'Etude des Lymphomes de l'Adulte. J Clin Oncol 2007;25:2825–32.

[9] Kiserud CE, Fosså A, Holte H, et al. Post-treatment parenthood in Hodgkin's lymphoma survivors. Br J Cancer 2007;96:1442–9.

[10] Fosså SD, Magelssen H. Fertility and reproduction after chemotherapy of adult cancer patients: malignant lymphoma and testicular cancer. Ann Oncol 2004;15(Suppl 4):259–65.

[11] Huddart RA, Norman A, Moynihan C, et al. Fertility, gonadal and sexual function in survivors of testicular cancer. Br J Cancer 2005;93:200–7.

[12] Brydøy M, Fosså SD, Klepp O, et al. Paternity following treatment for testicular cancer. J Natl Cancer Inst 2005;97:1580–8.

[13] Sjøborg KD, Vistad I, Myhr SS, et al. Pregnancy outcome after cervical cone excision: a case-control study. Acta Obstet Gynecol Scand 2007;86:423–8.

[14] Boss EA, van Golde RJ, Beerendonk CC, et al. Pregnancy after radical trachelectomy: a real option? Gynecol Oncol 2005;99(Suppl 1):152–6.

[15] Del Mastro L, Catzeddu T, Venturini M. Infertility and pregnancy after breast cancer: current knowledge and future perspectives. Cancer Treat Rev 2006;32:417–22.

[16] Cvancarova MS, Magelssen H, Fosså SD. Ten-year reproduction rates (10-RR) after cancer treatment: comparison between patients (cases) and the normal population (controls). J Clin Oncol 2007;25(185):9075.

[17] Magelssen H, Melve KK, Skjærven R, et al. Parenthood probability and pregnancy outcome in patients with a cancer diagnosis during adolescence and young adulthood. Hum Reprod 2008;23:461–5.

[18] Swerdlow AJ, Jacobs PA, Marks A, et al. Fertility, reproductive outcomes, and health of offspring, of patients treated for Hodgkin's disease: an investigation including chromosome examinations. Br J Cancer 1996;74:291–6.

[19] Stensheim H, Møller B, van Dijk T, et al. Cause-specific death in women diagnosed with cancer during pregnancy or lactation. Eur J Cancer 2007;5:160–1 [abstract no 1200].

[20] Magelssen H, Haugen TB, von Düring V, et al. Twenty years experience with semen cryopreservation in testicular cancer patients: who needs it? Eur Urol 2005;48:779–85.

[21] Oosterhuis JW, Looijenga LH. The biology of human germ cell tumours: retrospective speculations and new prospectives. Eur Urol 1993;23:245–50.

[22] Jacobsen KD, Olsen DR, Fosså K, et al. External beam abdominal radiotherapy in patients with seminoma stage I: field type, testicular dose, and spermatogenesis. Int J Radiat Oncol Biol Phys 1997;38:95–102.

[23] Jones WG, Fosså SD, Mead GM, et al. Randomized trial of 30 versus 20 Gy in the adjuvant treatment of stage I testicular seminoma: a report on Medical Research Council Trial TE18, European Organisation for the Research and Treatment of Cancer Trial 30942 (ISRCTN18525328). J Clin Oncol 2005;23:1200–8.

[24] Groll RJ, Warde P, Jewett MA. A comprehensive systematic review of testicular germ cell tumor surveillance. Crit Rev Oncol Hematol 2007;64:182–97.

[25] Donohue JP, Foster RS, Rowland RG, et al. Nerve-sparing retroperitoneal lymphadenectomy with preservation of ejaculation. J Urol 1990;144:287–91.

[26] Haukvik UK, Dieset I, Bjøro T, et al. Treatment-related premature ovarian failure as a long-term complication after Hodgkin's lymphoma. Ann Oncol 2006;17:1428–33.

[27] Gershenson DM, Miller AM, Champion VL, et al. Reproductive and sexual function after platinum-based chemotherapy in long-term ovarian germ cell tumor survivors: a Gynecologic Oncology Group Study. J Clin Oncol 2007;25:2792–7.

[28] Goto S, Ino K, Mitsui T, et al. Survival rates of patients with choriocarcinoma treated with chemotherapy without hysterectomy: effects of anticancer agents on subsequent births. Gynecol Oncol 2004;93:529–35.

[29] Heidenreich A, Weissbach L, Höltl W, et al. Organ sparing surgery for malignant germ cell tumor of the testis. J Urol 2001;166:2161–5.

[30] Agarwal A, Allamaneni SSR. Disruption of spermatogenesis by the cancer disease process. J Natl Cancer Inst Monogr 2005;34:9–12.

[31] Roberts JE, Oktay K. Fertility preservation: a comprehensive approach to the young woman with cancer. J Natl Cancer Inst Monogr 2005;34:57–9.

[32] Blumenfeld Z, Dann E, Avivi I, et al. Fertility after treatment for Hodgkin's disease. Ann Oncol 2002;13(Suppl 1):138–47.

[33] Simons JS, Carey MP. Prevalence of sexual dysfunctions: results from a decade of research. Arch Sex Behav 2001;30:177–219.

[34] Sjögren K, Fugl-Meyer AR. Sexual disabilities are not singularities. Int J Impot Res 2002;14:487–93.

[35] Pikler V, Winterowd C. Racial and body image differences in coping for women diagnosed with breast cancer. Health Psychol 2003;22:632–7.

[36] Katz A. The sound of silence: sexuality information for cancer patients. J Clin Oncol 2005;23:238–41.

[37] Basson R, Berman J, Burnett A, et al. Report on the international consensus development conference on female sexual dysfunction: definitions and classifications. J Urol 2000;163:888–93.

[38] Schover LR, von Eschenbach AC. Sexual and marital relationships after treatment for nonseminomatous testicular cancer. Urology 1985;25:251–5.

[39] Jonker-Pool G, Van de Wiel HB, Hoekstra HJ, et al. Sexual functioning after treatment for testicular cancer—review and meta-analysis of 36 empirical studies between 1975–2000. Arch Sex Behav 2001;30:55–74.

[40] Nazareth I, Lewin J, King M. Sexual dysfunction after treatment for testicular cancer: a systematic review. J Psychosom Res 2001;51:735–43.

[41] Laumann EO, Paik A, Rosen RC. Sexual dysfunction in the United States. Prevalence and predictors. JAMA 1999;281:537–44.

[42] Aass N, Grünfeld B, Kaalhus O, et al. Pre- and posttreatment sexual life in testicular cancer patients: a descriptive investigation. Br J Cancer 1993;67:1113–7.

[43] Incrocci L, Hop WCJ, Wijnmaalen A, et al. Treatment outcome, body image, and sexual functioning after orchiectomy and radiotherapy for stage I-II testicular seminoma. Int J Radiat Oncol Biol Phys 2002;53:1165–73.

[44] Jonker-Pool G, van Basten JP, Hoekstra HJ, et al. Sexual functioning after treatment for testicular cancer. Cancer 1997;80:454–64.

[45] Dahl AA, Bremnes R, Dahl O, et al. Is the sexual function compromised in long-term testicular cancer survivors? Eur Urol 2007;52:1438–47.

[46] Fobair P, Hoppe RT, Bloom J, et al. Psychosocial problems among survivors of Hodgkin's disease. J Clin Oncol 1986;4:805–14.

[47] Kornblith AB, Anderson J, Cella DF, et al. Comparison of psychosocial adaptation and sexual function of survivors of advanced Hodgkin disease treated by MOPP, ABVD, or MOPP alternating with ABVD. Cancer 1992;70:2508–16.

[48] Abrahamsen AF, Loge JH, Hannisdal E, et al. Socio-medical situation for long-term survivors of Hodgkin's disease: a survey of 459 patients treated at one institution. Eur J Cancer 1998;34:1865–70.

[49] Basson R. The female sexual response: a different model. J Sex Marital Ther 2000;26:51–65.

[50] Dorval M, Maunsell E, Taylor-Brown J, et al. Marital stability after breast cancer. J Natl Cancer Inst 1999;91:54–9.

[51] Kornblith AB, Ligibel J. Psychosocial and sexual functioning of survivors of breast cancer. Semin Oncol 2003;30:799–813.

[52] Wimberly SR, Carver CS, Laurenceau JP, et al. Perceived partner reactions to diagnosis and treatment of breast cancer: impact of psychosocial and psychosexual adjustment. J Consult Clin Psychol 2005;73:300–11.

[53] Hinnen C, Hagedoorn M, Sanderman R, et al. The role of distress, neuroticism and time since diagnosis in explaining support behaviors in partners of women with breast cancer: results of a longitudinal analysis. Psychooncology 2007;16:913–9.

[54] Ganz PA, Rowland JH, Desmond KA, et al. Life after breast cancer: understanding women's health-related quality of life and sexual functioning. J Clin Oncol 1998;16:501–14.

[55] Burwell SR, Case D, Kaelin C, et al. Sexual problems in younger women after breast cancer surgery. J Clin Oncol 2006;24:2815–21.

[56] Fobair P, Stewart SL, Chang S, et al. Body image and sexual problems in young women with breast cancer. Psychooncology 2006;15:579–94.

[57] Ganz PA, Kwan L, Stanton AL, et al. Quality of life at the end of primary treatment of breast cancer: first results from the moving beyond cancer randomized trial. J Natl Cancer Inst 2004;96:376–87.

[58] Baucom DH, Porter LS, Kirby JS, et al. Psychosocial issues confronting young women with breast cancer. Breast Dis 2006;23:103–13.

[59] Bloom JR, Stewart SL, Chang S, et al. Then and now: quality of life of young breast cancer survivors. Psychooncology 2004;13:147–60.

[60] Avis NE, Crawford S, Manuel J. Quality of life among younger women with breast cancer. J Clin Oncol 2005;23:3322–30.

[61] De Groot JM, Mah K, Fyles A, et al. The psychosocial impact of cervical cancer among affected women and their partners. Int J Gynecol Cancer 2005;15:918–25.

[62] Bergmark K, Avall-Lundqvist E, Dickman PW, et al. Vaginal changes and sexuality in women with a history of cervical cancer. N Engl J Med 1999;340:1383–9.

[63] Jensen PT, Groenvold M, Klee MC, et al. Longitudinal study of sexual function and vaginal changes after radiotherapy for cervical cancer. Int J Radiat Oncol Biol Phys 2003;56:937–49.

[64] Jensen PT, Groenvold M, Klee MC, et al. Early-stage cervical carcinoma, radical hysterectomy, and sexual function. A longitudinal study. Cancer 2004;100:97–106.

[65] Lindau ST, Gavrilova N, Anderson D. Sexual morbidity in very long term survivors of vaginal and cervical cancer: a comparison to national norms. Gynecol Oncol 2007;106:413–8.

[66] Vistad I, Fosså SD, Dahl AA. A critical review of patient-rated quality of life studies of long-term survivors of cervical cancer. Gynecol Oncol 2006;102:563–72.

[67] Frumovitz M, Sun CC, Schover LR, et al. Quality of life and sexual functioning in cervical cancer survivors. J Clin Oncol 2005;23:7428–36.

[68] Donovan KA, Taliaferro LA, Alvarez EM, et al. Sexual health in women treated for cervical cancer: characteristics and correlates. Gynecol Oncol 2007;104:428–34.

[69] Stewart DE, Wong F, Duff S, et al. "What doesn't kill you makes you stronger." An ovarian cancer survivor survey. Gynecol Oncol 2001;83:537–42.

[70] Carmack Taylor CL, Basen-Engquist K, Shinn EH, et al. Predictors of sexual functioning in ovarian cancer patients. J Clin Oncol 2004;22:881–9.

[71] Liavaag AH, Dørum A, Bjøro T, et al. A controlled study of sexual activity and functioning in epithelial ovarian cancer survivors. A therapeutic approach. Gynecol Oncol, in press.

Long-Term Cardiac and Pulmonary Complications of Cancer Therapy

Joachim Yahalom, MD[a],*, Carol S. Portlock, MD[b]

[a]Department of Radiation Oncology, Memorial Sloan-Kettering Cancer Center,
1275 York Avenue, New York, NY 10021, USA
[b]Department of Medicine, Memorial Sloan-Kettering Cancer Center,
1275 York Avenue, New York, NY 10021, USA

Many systemically administered chemotherapeutic and biologic agents may cause late cardiovascular complications [1,2]. Late cardiac effects are most commonly related to cancer treatment by anthracyclines, mitoxantrone, paclitaxel, docetaxel, and trastuzumab. The cardiotoxicity that results from mediastinal radiotherapy is discussed in detail. Pulmonary complications of chemotherapy and radiotherapy are discussed separately.

ANTHRACYCLINE-RELATED CARDIAC TOXICITY

Anthracyclines are a group of important potent drugs used in the treatment of many pediatric and adult malignancies. Anthracycline cardiomyopathy is characterized by a dose-dependent progressive decrease in systolic left ventricular function often leading to congestive heart failure. Abnormalities in left ventricular size and function measured by noninvasive testing can be detected before the development of overt congestive heart failure. Patients who have abnormal heart function following treatment with anthracyclines may or may not have clinical symptoms.

The delayed cardiomyopathy associated with anthracycline therapy presents clinically as classic congestive heart failure, including fatigue, shortness of breath, dyspnea on exertion, sinus tachycardia, S3 gallop rhythm, pedal edema/pleural effusions, and elevated jugular venous distention. These may be subtle at onset and progress gradually.

Anthracycline cardiomyopathy risk depends on the cumulative total dose [3]. At 450 mg/m^2 for doxorubicin there is a 5% risk, and for other anthracyclines this cumulative dose is: 900 mg/m^2 for daunorubicin, 935 mg/m^2 for epirubicin, and 223 mg/m^2 for idarubicin. Mediastinal irradiation that includes the heart, older (particularly >70 years) or younger (<15 years) age, coronary artery disease, other valvular or myocardial conditions, and hypertension are cofactors in cardiomyopathy risk. When administered concurrently,

*Corresponding author. E-mail address: yahalomj@mskcc.org (J. Yahalom).

0889-8588/08/$ – see front matter
doi:10.1016/j.hoc.2008.01.010

trastuzumab may potentiate anthracycline cardiotoxicity. Other agents with known cardiotoxic effects may be additive.

Cardiac dysfunction is established by comparing baseline with serial left ventricular function studies. Left ventricular ejection fraction (LVEF) may be measured by echocardiography or nuclear imaging and 50% or more is considered within the normal range. A low LVEF contraindicates the use of anthracyclines.

Typical findings on echocardiograms are left ventricular diastolic/systolic dysfunction and later septal wall motion dysfunction. The left ventricle is initially not enlarged or only moderately enlarged. Global hypokinesis and muscle wall thinning is seen with late cardiomyopathy. Sinus tachycardia, low voltage, poor R-wave progression, and nonspecific T wave changes are noted on EKG, but these are late findings and can be nonspecific.

In pediatrics, subclinical cardiomyopathy is more common than in adults at comparable doses, resulting in progressive loss of ventricular mass, reduced cardiac output, and restrictive cardiomyopathy. There does not seem to be a threshold cumulative dose below which left ventricular dysfunction is not seen [4–7].

Prevention of late cardiomyopathy requires the recognition of early dysfunction during chemotherapy. A decrease in ejection fraction, changes in diastolic function, and changes in troponins/brain natriuretic peptide have all been studied and are predictive in small series. The simplest is serial LVEF in susceptible patients, and discontinuing anthracycline with a significant decrease from baseline [8–10]. For doxorubicin, a repeat study should be performed at 200 mg/m^2, and all patients should have a follow-up study at 300 to 400 mg/m^2 and every 50 to 100 mg/m^2 thereafter.

Anthracycline strategies to reduce cardiovascular risk include: analogs, low-dose or infusional drug schedules, and the use of liposomal formulations [11,12]. Dexrazoxane decreases the risk for clinical cardiomyopathy with doxorubicin doses of 300 mg/m^2 or more [13]. Its role in upfront treatment regimens remains under investigation.

Anthracycline cardiomyopathy is managed like other causes of dilated cardiomyopathy with ACE inhibitors, β-blockers, and diuretics. These measures are palliative rather than curative and, unfortunately, the dysfunction may be progressive despite these agents. Cardiac transplantation provides the only curative option.

Selective cardiomyocyte apoptosis seems to play a major role in the development of anthracycline cardiomyopathy [14]. Cardiomyocyte metabolism of the anthracycline generates free radicals resulting in membrane lipid peroxidation with the consequent activation of the extrinsic and intrinsic apoptotic pathways, and cardiomyocyte intrinsic antioxidant defense is more limited than that of other organs.

Mitoxantrone is an anthracenedione, structurally related to the anthracyclines, and also causes a dose-related cardiomyopathy. Mitoxantrone cardiomyopathy is rarely seen before 100 mg/m^2 cumulative dose. LVEF should be monitored regularly thereafter and a total dose of 140 mg/m^2 should not be exceeded. Sequential use of doxorubicin followed by mitoxantrone raises cardiomyopathy risk [15]. The mechanism of cardiac damage with mitoxantrone is not fully understood.

TAXANES-RELATED CARDIAC TOXICITY
The taxanes, paclitaxel and docetaxel, are important antimicrotubule agents derived from the yew tree and their cardiotoxicity seems to be related to the taxane ring structural similarities to yew taxine.

Most of paclitaxel's cardiovascular effects are acute/subacute (asymptomatic bradycardia, hypersensitivity reactions, and life-threatening atrial or ventricular rhythm disturbances or conduction abnormalities in approximately 0.5% of patients) [16].

Congestive heart failure does not seem to be caused by paclitaxel, whereas it does seem to potentiate doxorubicin-associated cardiac dysfunction. The sequencing of paclitaxel and doxorubicin are critical in the development of cardiotoxicity [17–20] and is believed to be attributable to an interaction that results in reduced doxorubicin elimination and higher plasma levels [21]. Doxorubicin clearance is therefore paclitaxel schedule–dependent, occurring most prominently when paclitaxel immediately precedes doxorubicin or follows it by less than 1 hour. The taxane docetaxel does not seem to enhance doxorubicin cardiac dysfunction [22]. Although both taxanes increase toxic cardiomyocyte doxorubicinol production in vitro, only paclitaxel seems to be clinically cardiotoxic.

TRASTUZUMAB-RELATED CARDIAC TOXICITY
Trastuzumab is a humanized monoclonal antibody targeting p185^{HER2} (ErbB2 or HER2 receptor), a transmembrane receptor tyrosine kinase of the epidermal growth factor family. This receptor protein is overexpressed or amplified in 20% to 30% of breast cancer and trastuzumab is an important agent in the management of Her2-positive breast cancer.

Cardiac ErbB2 is essential for normal adult cardiac function; in a mouse model it has been shown that cardiac ErbB2-deficient mice develop a dilated cardiomyopathy beginning in the second postnatal month through adulthood. In addition, ErbB2-deficient cardiomyocytes are more susceptible to anthracycline toxicity [23,24].

Trastuzumab is specific for the human ErbB2 receptor and cannot be studied directly in mice. A two-hit model, in which hemodynamic overload or anthracycline exposure with trastuzumab promotes the development of cardiomyopathy, has been proposed [25]. In a recent prospective human study, trastuzumab preceding anthracycline-based adjuvant therapy revealed no cardiac toxicity, supporting this hypothesis [26].

Trastuzumab cardiotoxicity is well studied and a 4% to 10% incidence of cardiac dysfunction overall is reported [27,28]. Concurrent trastuzumab with paclitaxel or anthracycline-based regimens increases the incidence up to 25%. The degree of cardiac dysfunction is greatest with concurrent

trastuzumab/anthracycline as compared with trastuzumab/paclitaxel. Cardiomyopathy without recovery is seen in approximately half of affected trastuzumab/
anthracycline-treated patients, whereas most trastuzumab/paclitaxel-treated
patients recover. Older age, cumulative doxorubicin greater than or equal to
300 mg/m^2, and concurrent anthracycline are risk factors.

Like anthracycline cardiomyopathy, tachycardia and decrease in LVEF may
be early indicators with later progression to a full-blown cardiomyopathy. Unlike anthracyclines, trastuzumab cardiac toxicity is not antibody cumulative
dose dependent, and is more treatable and reversible [27]. Once reversed, trastuzumab can often be safely reintroduced with close monitoring.

Trastuzumab scheduling seems key to preventing cardiac toxicity. When
used before anthracycline, the cardiac stress signals that precipitate toxicity
may be eliminated [25]. Most importantly, avoidance of concurrent anthracycline exposure and identifying high-risk patients are essential.

RADIATION-RELATED CARDIOVASCULAR COMPLICATIONS

Radiotherapy of lymphomas involving the mediastinum, or radiation for lung
and breast cancers, may expose some (or rarely all) of the heart to potential
radiation damage. Of the most concern is the potential acceleration of coronary
artery disease that could lead to myocardial infarction or even sudden death.
Other long-term complications of cardiac irradiation include chronic pericarditis, valvular damage, arrhythmias, and conduction disturbances. Some data
suggest that anthracycline-induced congestive heart failure may be enhanced
in patients who received mediastinal irradiation in addition to anthracyclines.

Much of the information available on late complications of mediastinal radiation comes from children treated for Hodgkin lymphoma (HL). These patients received curative radiation treatment at a young age and thus provide
many years of follow-up that is required for a chronic disease to develop
[29]. Most of the studies reported in recent years on long-term cardiac complication include primarily patients who were treated in the 1960s through the
mid-1980s; this is the era when most patients who had HL, including children,
received radiation as a single modality. In those pioneer days of radiotherapy,
radiation in high doses was given to very large volumes (often including all or
most of the heart) using radiation technology that is now outdated [29].

Similar to the gradual progressive nature of anthracycline-related cardiac
toxicity that may remain latent to up to 20 years and is diagnosed only by special testing as a subclinical disease, radiation-related damage may be slow to develop and patients who have various degrees of damage remain asymptomatic
for years. Often more than one cardiac structure is affected and it is not unusual to find patients who have coronary artery disease and valvular disease
(clinical or subclinical).

Coronary Heart Disease in Patients Who Have Hodgkin Lymphoma

Experiments in laboratory animals [30–32], analysis of pathologic specimens
[33], clinical observations, and, in the 1990s, long-term risk analysis in large

series of patients treated for HL all indicate that mediastinal irradiation may facilitate the development of coronary heart disease (CHD) (Table 1) [35–41].

Stenosis at the origin of the coronary arteries seems to be a common finding for radiation-associated CHD [39,42,43]. After mediastinal irradiation, there is a greater likelihood for right coronary or left main or left anterior descending coronary artery lesions as opposed to circumflex lesions, which might be because the former vessels, particularly at their origin, receive more radiation [34].

The studies that analyzed the risk for mortality from myocardial infarction in patients who were treated for HL are summarized in Table 1. Although only approximately 1% to 2% of patients who had HL in these series died of myocardial infarction, the observed risk in all seven series was higher than expected.

The current involved-field radiotherapy concept, better fractionation schemes, modern equipment, and improved planning result in lower exposure of radiation to the coronary arteries and may have a lower risk for promoting CHD [44]. In a study by Boivin and colleagues [34], the relative risk for acute myocardial infarction was reduced from 6.33 for patients treated during the years 1940 to 1966 to 1.97 (with no significant difference from unity) for patients irradiated from 1967 to 1985.

Hancock and colleagues [35] analyzed the risk for cardiac disease in patients who had HL who were treated at Stanford from 1961 to 1991. In patients who

Table 1
Relative risk for mortality from myocardial infarction after mediastinal irradiation for Hodgkin lymphoma

Study	Center	Patients (n)	Lethal myocardial infarctions	Relative risk	95% CI
Boivin et al [34]	Multiple	4665	68	2.6	1.1–5.9
Hancock et al [35]	Stanford	2232	55	3.2	1.5–5.8
Henry-Amar et al [36]	European Organization for Treatment and Research on Cancer	1449	17	8.8	5.1–14.1
Mauch et al [37]	Joint Center for Radiation Therapy (Boston)	636	15[a]	2.2[a]	1.2–3.6
Glanzmann et al [38]	Zurich	352	8	4.2	1.8–8.3
Reinders et al [39]	Rotterdam	258	12[b]	5.3	2.7–9.3
Swerdlow et al [40]	Britain	7033	168	2.5	2.1–2.9

[a]Includes one patient who died of cardiomyopathy.
[b]Myocardial infarction or sudden death.

were irradiated before age 21 years the relative risk for death from acute myocardial infarction was 41.5 and the actuarial risk for fatal or nonfatal myocardial infarction at 22 years was 8.1%. Of note, all deaths in this study occurred in patients who received relatively high doses of radiation (42–45 Gy) to the mediastinum. When the Stanford analysis was extended to include 2232 patients of all age groups who had HL, the relative risk for death from acute myocardial infarction was 3.2 [35]. This study showed that patients younger than 20 years who received high-dose irradiation had the highest relative risk, that the risk decreases with increasing age, and that patients older than 50 years of age had no increased risk. These results contrast with data published by other investigators [34], however, suggesting an increased risk for acute myocardial infarction for the older age groups. The small number of patients in the Stanford study who received radiation doses of less than 30 Gy did not allow an adequate analysis of the dose effect. The average interval between HL treatment and death from acute myocardial infarction was 10.3 years, but risk was already significant during the first 5 years after treatment and remained elevated throughout the follow-up period (more than 20 years) [35].

Two European studies analyzed the risk for ischemic heart disease in patients who had HL who received standard fractions and dose (30–42 Gy) of mediastinal irradiation [38,39]. Both studies demonstrated an increase of ischemic heart disease after mediastinal irradiation. Of importance, a multivariate analysis of risk factors in the Rotterdam study showed that increasing age, gender (male), and a pretreatment cardiac medical history were significant for developing ischemic heart disease in irradiated patients [39]. In a study from Zurich, a detailed analysis of the effect of other CHD risk factors on the radiation-induced risk was performed. The study showed that, although the risk for CHD after irradiation increased by 4.2 for all patients, in irradiated female patients and in all irradiated patients who did not have other cardiovascular risk factors (smoking, hypertension, obesity, hypercholesterolemia, diabetes) the risk remained as expected in the normal population [38]. In a recent study of 1474 HL survivors treated mostly with radiation with or without chemotherapy, hypercholesterolemia was the most significant independent risk factor for developing CHD [41]. These data suggest that aggressive modification of CHD risk factors, such as hypercholesterolemia, is warranted in patients who received mediastinal radiation therapy or anthracycline-containing chemotherapy.

Although radiation was considered by some to be the only culprit in the induction of CHD in patients who had lymphoma and chemotherapy-alone regimens were supposed to avoid CHD, it was of surprise and concern to learn recently that anthracycline-containing regimens, such as ABVD (doxorubicin, bleomycin, vinblastine, dacarbazine) and R-CHOP (rituximab, cyclophosphamide, doxorubicin, vincristine, prednisone), even if given without radiotherapy, are associated with increased CHD risk [40,45]. Aviles studied 476 patients who had HL treated with anthracycline-containing chemotherapy and no radiation [45]. At a median follow-up of 11.5 years, 9% of patients who received ABVD had a clinical cardiac event and 7% had a cardiac-related death. The standard mortality ratio for cardiac death for patients who received doxorubicin was 46.4 (95% CI: 28.9–70.1) and the absolute excess risk (AER) was 39 [45].

The largest and most recent analysis of myocardial infarction (MI) mortality risk after treatment of HL is from a collaborative British cohort study of 7033 patients [40]. This study included 3590 patients who received radiotherapy without anthracyclines, 3052 patients who received chemotherapy with supradiaphragmatic radiation, and 1744 patients who received anthracycline regimens and no radiotherapy. For the whole group of HL survivors, the death from MI was significantly more than expected; SMR was 2.5 with an AER of 125.8. The risk was higher for males. The relative risk for death from MI decreased sharply with older age at first treatment, but as expected the AER increased with age. The 20-year cumulative risk for MI mortality for patients treated at age younger than 35 years was 1.8%. The risk for death during the first year after treatment was fourfold compared with the general population and it was higher for patients treated before 1980 [40].

Of particular concern are the new data regarding chemotherapy alone [40,45]. In the British study [40], the risk for death from MI was statistically significantly increased for patients who had received anthracyclines (SMR of 2.9) and especially those treated with ABVD (SMR of 9.5). These data remained significantly elevated for patients who received those chemotherapy regimens and no radiation therapy (SMR of 7.8). The authors suggested that the risk was particularly high for ABVD (compared with other doxorubicin-containing regimens) because ABVD alone was virtually always given for a full six cycles. The increased risk for patients treated with anthracyclines was primarily during the first year after treatment and the highest risk was in young patients (≤35 years). MI mortality risk was also significantly increased for treatment with vincristine with or without radiation [40].

Heart Disease Following Radiation of Breast Cancer

Long-term mortality data from three trials that randomized patients who had breast cancer to receive postmastectomy radiotherapy as opposed to no additional treatment demonstrated a higher incidence of cardiac death in the irradiated group [46–48]. The excess in mortality did not appear until after 10 years posttreatment [47,48]. In one study, the increase in mortality risk was significant only in women who were irradiated for tumors in the left breast. It was also increased in patients treated with orthovoltage irradiation, as opposed to those treated with more modern supervoltage equipment [48].

A recent study from the Netherlands of 4414 10-year breast cancer survivors who were treated from 1970 through 1986 recorded cardiovascular morbidity and mortality events [49,50]. It showed that radiation to the breast alone is not associated with increased risk for cardiovascular disease. Similar to other studies [51,52], it also documented that the increased risk for MI that was noted in patients treated before 1980 has disappeared with more recent radiation therapy techniques.

Techniques that reduce the risk for irradiating the coronary arteries have been developed; they include the prone breast technique [53] and use of three-dimensional CT planning and intensity-modulated radiation therapy [54]. Patients who have breast cancer irradiated with modern techniques are unlikely to receive a significant dose of radiation to the coronary arteries.

In patients who have breast cancer, conventional-dose doxorubicin-containing chemotherapy used as an adjuvant in combination with local-regional irradiation was not associated with a significant increase in the risk for cardiac events. Higher doses of adjuvant doxorubicin were associated with a three to fourfold increased risk for cardiac events, however. This finding seems to be especially true in patients treated with higher dose volumes of cardiac irradiation [55]. In one recent large-scale study, patients who had breast cancer who were treated with CMF (cyclophosphamide, methotrexate, 5-fluorouracil) and radiotherapy had a significantly higher risk for congestive heart failure compared with patients treated with radiotherapy alone [49].

Detection of Coronary Heart Disease in Asymptomatic Patients and Prevention Options

Monitoring and reduction of other contributing CHD risk factors in patients who received mediastinal irradiation should be part of the follow-up of patients who underwent mediastinal irradiation. The value of routine noninvasive or invasive cardiac studies in asymptomatic patients has not been fully determined, however [36,56–59]. In a recent screening study of 294 patients who received mediastinal radiation (median dose of 44 Gy) from 1960 to 1995, 21% of screened patients had abnormal ventricular images at rest [59]. During stress testing that included echocardiography and radionuclide perfusion 14% showed abnormalities in one or both tests. Based on these tests, 40 patients underwent coronary angiography and 55% of them (7% of the screened population) had 50% or greater stenosis. The risk for a cardiac event in those patients was significantly related to abnormal stress testing, older age, radiotherapy given in early period, and higher radiation therapy dose given to the mediastinum.

Early detection of CHD should be encouraged, particularly in patients irradiated with high radiation therapy dose (practiced mostly in the past) and those who have other CHD risk factors [56,57], because angioplastic or surgical intervention may be indicated in special anatomic or clinical situations [60]. Successful treatment of radiation-induced coronary disease with bypass surgery and with stenting or angioplasty has been reported [43,60,61]. In some cases, surgery may be technically difficult because of mediastinal and pericardial fibrosis [33].

RADIATION-INDUCED DELAYED PERICARDITIS

Late radiation-induced pericarditis that may occur between 4 months to several years after treatment is a relatively uncommon complication today [62,63].

Most cases of radiation-induced pericarditis and pericardial effusion resolve spontaneously, usually within 16 months. Rarely, patients who have delayed pericarditis progress within 5 to 10 years to develop symptomatic constriction requiring pericardiectomy. Occult constrictive pericarditis requires no surgical intervention and usually has a good prognosis.

RADIATION-INDUCED MYOCARDIAL DYSFUNCTION

When myocardial dysfunction is detected after standard-dose mediastinal irradiation, it is typically mild or subclinical [38,64,65]. Noninvasive studies using echocardiography and radionuclide angiography detected subtle left ventricular dysfunction in patients who had HL evaluated a few years after mediastinal irradiation [56]. A study of asymptomatic patients who were treated with mediastinal irradiation for HL at a young age showed reduced average left ventricular dimension and mass suggestive of restricted cardiomyopathy in 42% of patients [66]. Most patients who have abnormal ventricular function findings, however, do not have clinical heart failure [66]. The magnitude of the potential contribution of cardiac irradiation to the risk for doxorubicin-induced cardiomyopathy is not well established. Some data suggest potentiation of anthracycline-induced cardiotoxicity when combined with radiotherapy. Yet, the histopathologies of radiation heart disease and anthracycline heart disease are different, and the combined effects are probably additive rather than synergistic [65]. It was reported that doxorubicin-induced decrease in LVEF was aggravated with concurrent mediastinal irradiation [67,68]. In programs of combined modality therapy for HL that included relatively low doses of doxorubicin (up to 300 mg/m^2) and mediastinal irradiation of 20 to 40 Gy, no significant clinical myocardial dysfunction was detected [69].

Symptomatic myocardial dysfunction after a radiation dose that does not exceed 60 Gy is rare [51,52]. The few cases described with intractable heart failure had myocardial fibrosis as part of pancarditis, a generalized process with damage to all three layers of the heart. The hemodynamic pattern is usually of restrictive cardiomyopathy and is difficult to distinguish from constrictive pericarditis [64].

RADIATION-INDUCED VALVULAR DISEASE

Clinically significant valvular heart disease resulting from mediastinal irradiation is relatively uncommon [64]. Analysis of 635 patients treated for HL before the age of 21 years revealed 29 patients in whom new murmurs of indeterminate significance developed. Of those, 14 received mediastinal doses of 44 Gy or more, and 2 patients who received high-dose irradiation died of valvular heart disease [35]. When echocardiographic studies were performed in asymptomatic patients who had HL more than 7 years after mediastinal irradiation, valvular abnormalities were detected in 25% to 33% of the patients, although there was rarely any clinical significance. An echocardiographic study of 294 asymptomatic patients who received mediastinal irradiation disclosed moderate or severe regurgitation of the aortic valve in 5.0% of patients, of the mitral valve in 3.4%, and of the tricuspid valve in 1.4%. Four percent of the patients had aortic stenosis [70]. Valvular disease, particularly involving the aortic valve, increased with time after irradiation. Of 73 asymptomatic patients evaluated more than 20 years after mediastinal irradiation, 60% had mild or more aortic regurgitation and 16% had aortic stenosis. Radiation dose, volumes, and technique of radiation delivery have markedly changed over the last 3 decades, and the lower prevalence of valvular disease in patients treated at less than 20 years may reflect those changes [71]. In a retrospective study of 415 patients who were irradiated from 1962 to 1998, 6.2% of patients developed clinically significant valvular dysfunction at a median of 22 years [68]. Of interest is a report from Norway that showed a significantly higher risk for cardiopulmonary complications for female subjects after radiation for HL [44,72]. The mean interval from irradiation to detection of valvular disease in asymptomatic and symptomatic patients was 11.5 and 16.5 years, respectively [73]. Patients who received mediastinal radiotherapy and an anthracycline-containing chemotherapy had significantly more valvular disorders than patients receiving radiation therapy with no anthracyclines [41].

LATE CHEMOTHERAPY- OR RADIATION-INDUCED PULMONARY TOXICITY

Although many chemotherapeutic agents and radiation of the lungs may cause acute pulmonary toxicity, chronic pulmonary complications in cancer survivors are relatively rare. Bleomycin, the chemotherapy drug notorious for acute pneumonitis, is the most-studied agent. It is often used for germ cell tumors and for Hodgkin and non-Hodgkin lymphomas. Risk factors for bleomycin toxicity are bleomycin cumulative dose, age, smoking, renal dysfunction, mediastinal radiotherapy, and administration of oxygen [74,75]. Most patients who have acute bleomycin-induced pneumonitis recover with discontinuation of the drug or corticosteroid treatment. Only a minority progress to pulmonary fibrosis [74].

Radiation pneumonitis has been reported mostly in patients irradiated for lung cancer, Hodgkin or non-Hodgkin lymphoma involving the mediastinum, breast cancer, or other tumors involving the thorax. In patients who received radiotherapy for lung cancer, the risk for radiation pneumonitis is in the range of 5% to 15%. The risk is increased with concomitant chemotherapy, previous history of lung irradiation, and withdrawal of corticosteroids [76]. In a retrospective multivariate analysis of a large group of patients who had both chemotherapy and radiation, higher daily radiation fractions and the total radiation dose were associated with a significantly higher risk for pneumonitis. The overall risk was 7.8% [77].

The risk for pneumonitis after radiation for Hodgkin lymphoma involving the mediastinum or after radiation for breast cancer is markedly lower than in patients who have lung cancer. With modern techniques, lower doses, and conformation of the radiation field to the postchemotherapy residual mass, the risk for posttreatment subacute pneumonitis is less than 3% in lymphomas and less than 1% in breast cancer. The vast majority of patients who experience posttreatment radiation pneumonitis have a self-limited course with complete resolution of the process and the clinical symptoms. Patients who develop acute bleomycin pneumonitis or subacute radiation pneumonitis are followed with pulmonary function tests and most show significant improvement over time [78].

References

[1] Jones RL, Swanton C, Ewer M. Anthracycline cardiotoxicity. Expert Opin Drug Saf 2006; 5(6):791–809.

[2] Jones RL, Ewer MS. Cardiac and cardiovascular toxicity of nonanthracycline anticancer drugs [review]. Expert Rev Anticancer Ther 2006;6(9):1249–69.

[3] Keefe DL. Anthracycline-induced cardiomyopathy. Semin Oncol 2001;28(12):2–7.

[4] Giantris A, Abdurrahman L, Hinkle A, et al. Anthracycline-induced cardiotoxicity in children and young adults. Crit Rev Oncol Hematol 1998;27(1):53–68.

[5] Massin MM, Dresse MF, Schmitz V, et al. Acute arrhythmogenicity of first-dose chemotherapeutic agents in children. Med Pediatr Oncol 2002;39:93–8.

[6] Kremer LCM, van der Pal HJH, Offringa M, et al. Frequency and risks factors of subclinical cardiotoxicity after anthracycline therapy in children: a systematic review. Ann Oncol 2002;13:819–29.

[7] Lipshultz SE, Lipsitz SR, Sallan SE, et al. Chronic progressive cardiac dysfunction years after doxorubicin therapy for childhood acute lymphoblastic leukemia. J Clin Oncol 2005; 23(12):2629–36.

[8] Nousiainen T, Jantunen E, Vanninen E, et al. Early decline in left ventricular ejection fraction predicts doxorubicin cardiotoxicity in lymphoma patients. Br J Cancer 2002;86:1697–700.

[9] Mitani I, Jain D, Joska TM, et al. Doxorubicin cardiotoxicity: prevention of congestive heart failure with serial cardiac function monitoring with equilibrium radionuclide angiocardiography in the current era. J Nucl Cardiol 2003;10:132–9.

[10] Suter TM, Meier B. Detection of anthracycline-induced cardiotoxicity: is there light at the end of the tunnel? Ann Oncol 2002;13(5):647–9.

[11] van Dalen EC, Michiels EM, Caron HN, et al. Different anthracycline derivates for reducing cardiotoxicity in cancer patients. Cochrane Database Syst Rev 2006;(4):CD005006.

[12] van Dalen CD, van der Pal HJH, Caron HN, et al. Different dosage schedules for reducing cardiotoxicity in cancer patients receiving anthracycline chemotherapy [review]. Cochrane Database Syst Rev 2006;(4):CD005008.

[13] Swain SM, Whaley FS, Gerber MC, et al. Cardioprotection with dexrazoxane for doxorubicin-containing therapy in advanced breast cancer. J Clin Oncol 1997;15:1318–32.

[14] Minotti G, Menna P, Salvatorelli E, et al. Anthracyclines: molecular advances and pharmacologic developments in antitumor activity and cardiotoxicity [review]. Pharmacol Rev 2004;56(2):185–229.

[15] Clark GM, Tokaz LK, Von Hoff DD, et al. Cardiotoxicity in patients treated with mitoxantrone on Southwest Oncology Group phase II protocols. Cancer Treatment Symposia 1984;3: 25–30.

[16] Arbuck SG, Strauss H, Rowinsky E, et al. A reassessment of cardiac toxicity associated with Taxol. J Natl Cancer Inst Monogr 1993;15:117–30.

[17] Giordano SH, Booser DJ, Murray JL, et al. A detailed evaluation of cardiac toxicity: a phase II study of doxorubicin and one- or three-hour-infusion paclitaxel in patients with metastatic breast cancer. Clin Cancer Res 2002;8:3360–8.

[18] Biganzoli L, Cufer T, Bruning P, et al. Doxorubicin-paclitaxel: a safe regimen in terms of cardiac toxicity in metastatic breast carcinoma patients. Results from a European organization for research and treatment of cancer multicenter trial. Cancer 2003;97: 40–5.

[19] Gianni L, Dombernowsky P, Sledge G, et al. Cardiac function following combination therapy with paclitaxel and doxorubicin: an analysis of 657 women with advanced breast cancer. Ann Oncol 2001;12:1067–73.

[20] Tan-Chiu E, Yothers G, Romond E, et al. Assessment of cardiac dysfunction in a randomized trial comparing doxorubicin and cyclophosphamide followed by paclitaxel, with or without trastuzumab as adjuvant therapy in node-positive, human epidermal growth factor receptor 2-overexpressing breast cancer: NSABP B-31. J Clin Oncol 2005;23(31):7811–9.

[21] Holmes FA, Madden T, Newman RA, et al. Sequence-dependent alteration of doxorubicin pharmacokinetic by paclitaxel in a phase I study of paclitaxel and doxorubicin in patients with metastatic breast cancer. J Clin Oncol 1996;14(10):2713–21.

[22] Chan S, Friedrichs K, Noel D, et al. Prospective randomized trial of docetaxel versus doxorubicin in patients with metastatic breast cancer. J Clin Oncol 1999;17(8):2341–54.

[23] Crone SA, Zhao YY, Fan L, et al. ErbB2 is essential in the prevention of dilated cardiomyopathy. Nat Med 2002;8(5):459–65.

[24] Ozcelik C, Erdmann B, Pilz B, et al. Conditional mutation of the ErbB2 (HER2) receptor in cardiomyocytes leads to dilated cardiomyopathy. Proc Natl Acad Sci U S A 2002; 99(13):8880–5.

[25] Chien KR. Herceptin and the heart—a molecular modifier of cardiac failure. N Engl J Med 2006;354(8):789–90.

[26] Joensuu H, Kellokumpu-Lehtinen PL, Bono P, et al. Adjuvant docetaxel or vinorelbine with or without trastuzumab for breast cancer. N Engl J Med 2006;354(8):809–20.

[27] Smith K, Dang C, Seidman AD. Cardiac dysfunction associated with trastuzumab. Expert Opin Drug Saf 2006;5(5):619–29.

[28] Seidman A, Hudis C, Pierri MK, et al. Cardiac dysfunction in the trastuzumab clinical trials experience. J Clin Oncol 2002;20(5):1215–21.

[29] Carver JR, Shapiro CL, Ng A, et al. American Society of Clinical Oncology Clinical Evidence Review on the Ongoing Care of Adult Cancer Survivors: cardiac and pulmonary late effects. J Clin Oncol 2007;25:3991–4008.

[30] Amronim GD, Solomon RD. Production of arteriosclerosis in the rabbit: a quantitative assessment. Arch Pathol 1965;75:219.

[31] Gold H. Production of arteriosclerosis in the rat: effect of X-ray and high-fat diet. Arch Pathol 1961;71:268.

[32] Artom C, Lofton HB, Clarkson TB. Ionizing radiation atherosclerosis and lipid metabolism in pigeons. Radiat Res 1965;26:165.

[33] McEniery PT, Dorosti K, Schiavone WA, et al. Clinical and angiographic features of coronary artery disease after chest irradiation. Am J Cardiol 1987;60:1020.

[34] Boivin JF, Hutchison GB, Lubin JH, et al. Coronary artery disease mortality in patients treated for Hodgkin's disease. Cancer 1992;69:1241.

[35] Hancock SL, Tucker MA, Hoppe RT. Factors affecting late mortality from heart disease after treatment of Hodgkin's disease. JAMA 1993;270:1949.

[36] Henry-Amar M, Hayat M, Meerwaldt JH. Causes of death after therapy for early stage Hodgkin's disease entered on EORTC protocols. Int J Radiat Oncol Biol Phys 1990;19: 1155.

[37] Mauch P, Kalish L, Marcus KC, et al. Long-term survival in Hodgkin's disease. Cancer J Sci Am 1995;1:33.

[38] Glanzmann C, Kaufmann P, Jenni R, et al. Cardiac risk after mediastinal irradiation for Hodgkin's disease. Radiother Oncol 1998;46:51.

[39] Reinders JG, Heijmen BJ, Olofsen-van Acht MJ, et al. Ischemic heart disease after mantlefield irradiation for Hodgkin's disease in long-term follow-up. Radiother Oncol 1999;51:35.

[40] Swerdlow AJ, Higgins CD, Smith P, et al. Myocardial infarction mortality risk after treatment for Hodgkin disease: a collaborative British cohort study. J Natl Cancer Inst 2007;99: 206–14.

[41] Aleman BM, van del Belt-Dusebout AW, De Bruin M, et al. Late cardiotoxicity after treatment for Hodgkin lymphoma. Blood 2007;109:1878–86.

[42] Handler CE, Livesey S, Lawton PA. Coronary ostial stenosis after radiotherapy: angioplasty or coronary artery surgery? Br Heart J 1989;61:208.

[43] Orzan F, Brusca A, Conte MR, et al. Severe coronary artery disease after radiation therapy of the chest and mediastinum: clinical presentation and treatment. Br Heart J 1993;69:496.

[44] Lund MB, Kongerud J, Boe J, et al. Cardiopulmonary sequelae after treatment for Hodgkin's disease: increased risk in females? Ann Oncol 1996;7:257.

[45] Aviles A, Neri N, Nambo MJ, et al. Late cardiac toxicity secondary to treatment in Hodgkin's disease. A study comparing doxorubicin, epirubicin and mitoxantrone in combined therapy. Leuk Lymphoma 2005;46:1023–8.

[46] Host H, Brennhoud IO, Loeb M. Post-operative radiotherapy in breast cancer: long-term results from the Oslo study. Int J Radiat Oncol Biol Phys 1986;12:727.

[47] Jones JM, Ribeiro GG. Mortality patterns over 34 years of breast cancer patients in a clinical trial of post-operative radiotherapy. Clin Radiol 1989;40:204.

[48] Haybittle JL, Brinkley D, Houghton J, et al. Postoperative radiotherapy and late mortality: evidence from the Cancer Research Campaign trial for early breast cancer. BMJ 1989;298:1611.

[49] Hooning MJ, Berthe A, Aleman MP, et al. Long-term risk of cardiovascular disease in 10-year survivors of breast cancer. J Natl Cancer Inst 2007;99:365–75.

[50] Giordano SH, Hortobagyi GN. Local recurrence of cardiovascular disease: pay now or later. J Natl Cancer Inst 2007;99:340–1.

[51] Darby SC, McGale P, Taylor CW, et al. Long-term mortality from heart disease and lung cancer after radiotherapy breast cancer: prospective cohort study of about 300,000 women in US SEE registries. Lancet Oncol 2005;6:539–40.

[52] Giordano SH, Juo YF, Freeman JL, et al. Risk of cardiac death after adjuvant radiotherapy for breast cancer. J Natl Cancer Inst 2005;97:406–7.

[53] Stegman LD, Beal KP, Hunt MA, et al. Long-term clinical outcomes of whole-breast irradiation delivered in the prone position. Int J Radiat Oncol Biol Phys 2007;68:73–81.

[54] Landau D, Adams EJ, Webb S, et al. Cardiac avoidance in breast radiotherapy: a comparison of simple shielding techniques with intensity-modulated radiotherapy. Radiother Oncol 2001;60:247.

[55] Shapiro CL, Hardenbergh PH, Gelman R, et al. Cardiac effects of adjuvant doxorubicin and radiation therapy in breast cancer patients. J Clin Oncol 1998;16:3493.

[56] Savage DE, Constine LS, Schwartz RG, et al. Radiation effects on left ventricular function and myocardial perfusion in long-term survivors of Hodgkin's disease. Int J Radiat Oncol Biol Phys 1990;19:721.

[57] Pierga JY, Maunoury C, Valette H, et al. Follow-up thallium-201 scintigraphy after mantle field radiotherapy for Hodgkin's disease. Int J Radiat Oncol Biol Phys 1993;25:871.

[58] Pihkala J, Happonen JM, Virtanen K, et al. Cardiopulmonary evaluation of exercise tolerance after chest irradiation and anticancer chemotherapy in children and adolescents. Pediatrics 1995;95:755.

[59] Piovaccari G, Ferretti RM, Prati F, et al. Cardiac disease after chest irradiation for Hodgkin's disease: incidence in 108 patients with long follow-up. Int J Cardiol 1995;49:39.

[60] Reber D, Birnbaum DE, Tollenaere P. Heart disease following mediastinal irradiation: surgical management. Eur J Cardiothorac Surg 1995;9:202–5.

[61] Van Son JA, Noyez L, van Asten WN. Use of internal mammary artery in myocardial revascularization after mediastinal irradiation. J Thorac Cardiovasc Surg 1992;104:1539.

[62] Adams MJ, Lipshutz SE, Schwartz C, et al. Radiation-associated cardiovascular disease: manifestations and management. Semin Radiat Oncol 2003;13:346.

[63] Ruckdeschel JC, Chang P, Martin RG, et al. Radiation-related pericardial effusions in patients with Hodgkin's disease. Medicine 1975;54:245.

[64] Arsenian MA. Cardiovascular sequelae of therapeutic thoracic radiation. Prog Cardiovasc Dis 1991;33:299.

[65] Lagrange JL, Darcourt J, Benoliel J, et al. Acute cardiac effects of mediastinal irradiation: assessment by radionuclide angiography. Int J Radiat Oncol Biol Phys 1992;22:897.

[66] Adams MJ, Lipsitz SR, Colan SD, et al. Cardiovascular status in long-term survivors of Hodgkin's disease treated with chest radiotherapy. J Clin Oncol 2004;22:3139–48.

[67] Clements IP, Davis BJ, Wiseman GA. Systolic and diastolic cardiac dysfunction early after the initiation of doxorubicin therapy: significance of gender and concurrent mediastinal radiation. Nucl Med Commun 2002;23:521.

[68] Hequet Q, Le QH, Moullet I, et al. Subclinical late cardiomyopathy after doxorubicin therapy for lymphoma in adults. J Clin Oncol 2004;22:1864–71.

[69] Glanzmann C, Huguenin P, Lutolf UM, et al. Cardiac lesions after mediastinal irradiation for Hodgkin's disease. Radiother Oncol 1994;30:43.

[70] Heidenreich PA, Hancock SL, Lee BK, et al. Asymptomatic cardiac disease following mediastinal irradiation. J Am Coll Cardiol 2003;42:743.

[71] Byrd BF III, Mendes LA. Cardiac complications of mediastinal radiotherapy. The other side of the coin. J Am Coll Cardiol 2003;42:750.

[72] Gustavsson A, Eskilsson J, Landberg T, et al. Late cardiac effects after mantle radiotherapy in patients with Hodgkin's disease. Ann Oncol 1990;1:355.

[73] Carlson RG, Mayfield WR, Normann S, et al. Radiation-associated valvular disease. Chest 1991;99:538.

[74] Sleijfer S. Bleomycin-induced pneumonitis. Chest 2001;120:617–24.

[75] O'Sullivan JM, Huddar RA, Norman AR, et al. Predicting the risk of bleomycin lung toxicity in patients with germ-cell tumors. Ann Oncol 2003;14:91–6.

[76] McDonald S, Rubin P, Phillips TL, et al. Injury to the lung from cancer therapy: clinical syndromes, measurable endpoints, and potential scoring systems. Int J Radiat Oncol Biol Phys 1995;31:1187–203.

[77] Roach M III, Gandara DR, Yuo HS, et al. Radiation pneumonitis following combined modality therapy for lung cancer: analysis of prognostic factors. J Clin Oncol 1995;13:2606–12.

[78] Hirsch A, Vander Els N, Straus DJ, et al. Effect of ABVD chemotherapy with and without mantle or mediastinal irradiation on pulmonary function and symptoms in early-stage Hodgkin's disease. J Clin Oncol 1996;14:1297–305.

Promoting a Healthy Lifestyle Among Cancer Survivors

Wendy Demark-Wahnefried, PhD, RD[a],*, Lee W. Jones, PhD[b]

[a]Department of Behavioral Science, The University of Texas–MD Anderson Cancer Center, 1155 Herman P. Pressler, CPPB3.3245, Houston, TX 77030, USA
[b]Department of Surgery, Duke University Medical Center, Box 3624 DUMC, Durham, NC 27710, USA

This year, roughly 1.6 million people in the United States and Canada will be diagnosed with cancer [1,2]. Given advances in early detection and treatment, two thirds of those diagnosed with this disease can expect to be alive in 5 years [1]. These individuals will join the ever-expanding numbers of cancer survivors who now comprise 3% to 4% of the North American population [3]. Although these statistics are encouraging, it is important to acknowledge that the impact of cancer is significant and associated with several long-term health and psychosocial sequelae [4–17]. In addition to risk for recurrence, data clearly show that compared with general age- and race-matched populations, cancer survivors are at greater risk for developing second malignancies, cardiovascular disease, diabetes, osteoporosis, and functional decline [4–17]. These comorbid conditions and competing causes of death are believed to result from cancer treatment, genetic predisposition, or common lifestyle factors [12,13,17].

In two recent Institute of Medicine (IOM) reports the numerous health issues of cancer survivors were summarized, and the potential benefits of lifestyle modifications were reviewed [18,19]. Also during this period of time, the American Cancer Society reissued its guide for Informed Choices on Nutrition and Physical Activity During and After Cancer Treatment [20,21]. Taken together, these reports serve as resources for health care providers, patient advocates, and other stakeholders to improve the health and well-being of this rapidly expanding and high risk population (Boxes 1 and 2 for reproduced diet and physical activity guidelines published within the American Cancer Society report). This article reviews these recommendations in light of more recent advances, with the following topic areas addressed: strength of evidence for

This work was supported by Grant No. CA106919 (WDW) and CA122143 (WDW, LWJ) from the National Institutes of Health, and MD Anderson Cancer Center (WDW).

*Corresponding author. E-mail address: wdemarkw@mdanderson.org (W. Demark-Wahnefried).

Box 1: American Cancer Society guidelines on nutrition and physical activity for cancer prevention

Maintain a healthy weight throughout life

- Balance caloric intake with physical activity
- Avoid excessive weight gain throughout the lifecycle
- Achieve and maintain a healthy weight if currently overweight or obese

Adopt a physically active lifestyle

- Adults: engage in at least 30 minutes of moderate-to-vigorous physical activity, above usual activities, on 5 or more days of the week; 45 to 60 minutes of intentional physical activity are preferable
- Children and adolescents: engage in at least 60 min/day of moderate-to-vigorous physical activity at least 5 days per week

Consume a healthy diet, with an emphasis on plant sources

- Choose foods and beverages in amounts that help achieve and maintain a healthy weight
- Eat five or more servings of a variety of vegetables and fruits each day
- Choose whole grains in preference to processed (refined) grains
- Limit consumption of processed and red meats

If you drink alcoholic beverages, limit consumption

- Drink no more than one drink per day for women or two per day for men

From Doyle C, Kushi LH, Byers T, et al. Nutrition and physical activity during and after cancer treatment: an American Cancer Society guide for informed choices. CA Cancer J Clin 2006;56:323–53; with permission.

recommendations in areas of weight management, diet, exercise, and smoking cessation; and current evidence examining the efficacy of various intervention approaches to promote health behavior changes among adult cancer survivors. To this end, an updated search of literature published on adult cancer survivors within the past 2 years was performed using CancerLit, PubMed, and Medline databases and using the following search terms: cancer survivors or neoplasms/survivor cross-referenced with MeSH terms of life style, health behavior, cardiovascular training, rehabilitation, physical fitness, physical activity, exercise, body weight, obesity, weight loss, diet, nutrition, tobacco, smoking cessation, and intervention studies. Relevant articles were then hand searched for pertinent previously published papers. Because prospective intervention studies offer the strongest evidence regarding potential benefit, key elements of recent lifestyle intervention trials that have health-related end points have been excerpted and included in Table 1.

LIFESTYLE CONCERNS FOR CANCER SURVIVORS

Weight Management

Positive and negative energy balance are dual concerns in cancer populations. As noted in both the IOM and American Cancer Society reports [18–20], as

---

Box 2: Exercise prescription guidelines for cancer survivors after completion of primary treatment

Low-intensity (light effort) endurance exercise
- 20%–39% of $HR_{reserve}$; 40%–50% VO_{2peak}; RPE of 10–11; 2–4 METs
- 45–60 min/day (total exercise minutes can be accumulated by performing short bouts of light-intensity endurance exercise throughout the day)
- 5–7 days of week
- Gardening, carrying groceries, raking lawn

Moderate-intensity (moderate effort) endurance exercise
- 40%–59% of $HR_{reserve}$; 60%–75% VO_{2peak}; RPE of 12–13; 4–6 METs
- 20–60 min/day (total exercise minutes can be accumulated by performing short bouts of moderate-intensity endurance exercise throughout the day)
- 3–5 days of week
- Brisk walking ($\geq$2.5–4 mph), swimming, cycling

Vigorous-intensity (strenuous effort) endurance exercise
- 60%–84% of $HR_{reserve}$; $\geq$75% VO_{2peak}; RPE of 14–16; 6–8 METs
- 20–45 min/day (total exercise minutes can be accumulated by performing short bouts of vigorous-intensity endurance exercise throughout the day)
- 3–5 days of week
- Jogging ($\geq$5 mph), vigorous swimming, vigorous cycling

Progressive resistance exercise (weight-bearing)
- One to two sets (8–12 repetitions each) of 8–10 large-muscle group resistance exercises at moderate intensity
- 2–3 nonconsecutive days of week

Flexibility and stretching exercise (weight-bearing)
- Gentle reaching, bending, and stretching of the large muscle groups
- Hold each stretch for 20–30 seconds; perform each stretch at least twice

Calculations: $HR_{reserve}$ = maximal heart rate (HR_{max}) minus resting heart rate (HR_{rest}). Multiply $HR_{reserve}$ by 0.20 to 0.84 to obtain target heart rate for desired intensity of exercise.

Abbreviations: HR, heart rate; METs, metabolic equivalent; RPE, rate of perceived exertion; VO_{2peak}, peak oxygen consumption (mL.kg.min^{-1}).
Adapted from Jones LW, Demark-Wahnefried W. Diet, exercise, and complementary therapies after primary treatment for cancer. Lancet Oncol 2006;7(12):1017–26; with permission.

critical as anorexia and cachexia are to cancer care, for most cancer survivors obesity and overweight are problems that are far more prevalent [20–23]. Obesity is a well-established risk factor for cancers of the breast (postmenopausal), colon, kidney (renal cell), esophagus (adenocarcinoma), and endometrium [24]; a high proportion of cancer survivors are overweight or obese at the time of diagnosis. Furthermore, increased premorbid body weight or body weight at the time of diagnosis has been associated with overall and cancer-specific

Table 1
Diet and exercise intervention trials employing cancer-specific or general health outcomes (March 2006–October 2007)

Authors	Site	Sample	Age	Design	Intervention	Frequency/ intensity/duration	Results
Dietary interventions							
Chlebowski et al [54]	Breast	2437 post-menopausal patients diagnosed with localized disease within 12 months	48–79 years Mean = 58.5 years	RCT	Low fat, nutrient adequate diet (<15% of total energy) versus a nutrient adequate diet	5 year median follow-up	Overall, patients assigned to the low fat diet had significant reductions in recurrence (HR= 0.76; 95% CI: 0.6-0.98); though this effect was limited to patients who had ER-receptor disease HR=0.58; 95% CI: 0.37-0.91); and not patients with ER+ disease (HR=0.85; 95% CI: 0.63-1.14).

Pierce et al [60]	Breast	3088 pre- & post-menopausal patients diagnosed with stage I-IIIA disease within 4 years	18–70 years Mean = 53 years	RCT	Very high V&F (5+ daily servings of vegetables, 3+ daily servings of fruit +16 oz. of vegetable juice/day), low fat (15%–20% of energy) and high fiber (30 g/day) diet versus standard instruction on 5+ daily servings of V&F	7.3 year mean follow-up	No significant differences in rates of breast cancer recurrence found between study arms (HR=.96 95% CI: 0.8-1.14).
Exercise interventions De Backer et al [65]	Mixed	57 patients who had received chemotherapy for lymphoma, breast, gynecologic, testicular, or colorectal cancer	24 to 73	Pre-Post	Supervised high-intensity resistance training program	1 to 2 times/wk of 6 exercises at 65% to 80% of one-repetition maximum for 18 weeks	Statistically significant ↑ in muscle strength, exercise capacity (VO$_{2peak}$), and QOL

(continued on next page)

Table 1
(continued)

Authors	Site	Sample	Age	Design	Intervention	Frequency/intensity/duration	Results
Daley et al [66]	Breast cancer	108 operable breast cancer patients who had received adjuvant therapy who were 12–36 mths post treatment	Mean age ~ 50	RCT	Participants were randomized to 1 of 3 groups: (1) Supervised aerobic exercise training (2) Supervised placebo-Exercise (3) Usual Care	A Aerobic Exercise Group: 3x/wk @ 65% to 85% of heart rate max Placebo-Exercise Group: Light-intensity stretching/conditioning 3x/wk for 18 weeks	Statistically significant ↑ QOL & aerobic fitness favoring aerobic exercise versus usual care. Indices of psychosocial health improved for both intervention groups
Herrero et al [67]	Breast cancer	16 operable breast cancer survivors who had completed primary adjuvant therapy	Mean age ~ 50	RCT	Supervised combined aerobic and resistance training program	3x, 90 minute sessions/wk at a moderate intensity for 8 weeks	Statistically significant ↑ QOL, VO_{2peak}, and muscle strength

| Milne et al [68] | Breast cancer | 58 operable breast cancer patients within 2 years of completing primary therapy | Mean age ~ 50 | RCT | Supervised combined aerobic and resistance training program | Aerobic training (20 mins in duration) & resistance training (12 different exercises) performed 3x/wk for 12 weeks. No intensity was provided | Statistically significant ↑ overall QOL, subcomponents of QOL that favored the exercise group. No significant between group ↑ in aerobic fitness and muscle strength |
| Nikander et al [69] | Breast cancer | 30 operable breast cancer patients within 6 months of chemotherapy completion | 41 to 65 | RCT | Supervised and home-based aerobic exercise training | 1x/wk & home-based exercise 2x/wk at a moderate intensity for 12 weeks | Significant between-group differences in several physical performance outcomes. |

(continued on next page)

Table 1
(continued)

Authors	Site	Sample	Age	Design	Intervention	Frequency/intensity/duration	Results
Schneider et al [70]	Breast cancer	96 operable breast cancer patients who had completed adjuvant therapy	Mean age ~ 50	Pre-Post	Supervised aerobic-based exercise sessions	Exercise sessions performed 2 to 3x/wk at 40% to 70% of heart rate reserve for 24 weeks	Significant within group improvements in blood pressure, heart rate, cardiopulmonary fitness (predicted VO_{2max}), pulmonary function. Improvements were also observed for several psychosocial outcomes

Schneider et al [71]	Mixed	37 male cancer survivors who had received treatment for prostate, colon, Hodgkin's, lung cancer	Mean age ~ 64	Pre-Post	Supervised aerobic-based exercise sessions	Exercise sessions performed 2 to 3x/wk at 40% to 70% of heart rate reserve for 12 weeks	Significant within group improvements in, heart rate and cardiopulmonary fitness (predicted VO_{2max}). Improvements were also observed for several psychosocial outcomes

Multicomponent interventions (diet and exercise)

Demark-Wahnefried et al [53]	Breast and prostate	182 elderly breast and prostate cancer survivors diagnosed within the 18 months	Age 65+, Mean age 72 years	RCT	Home-based, telephone counseling – mailed material intervention on diet and exercise versus telephone counseling and mailed materials on general health topics	Telephone counseling delivered every two weeks for 24 weeks	As compared with attention controls, Intervention participants significant improved diet quality (−2.9 versus +2.2; $P = .003$); trends were observed in physical activity energy expenditure (−400 versus + 111 kcal/week) and physical functioning (−0.5 versus +3.1)

mortality for cancers of the breast, esophagus, colon and rectum, cervix, uterus, liver, gallbladder, stomach, pancreas, prostate, kidney, non-Hodgkin's lymphoma, and multiple myeloma, and all cancers combined [25–31]. Finally, additional weight gain is common during or after treatment for various cancers, and has been found to reduce quality of life (QOL) and exacerbate risk for functional decline, comorbidity, and perhaps even cancer recurrence and cancer-related death [19,20,32,33]. Although studies exploring the relationship between postdiagnosis weight gain and disease-free survival have been somewhat inconsistent [22,32,34,35], one of the largest studies (N = 5204) by Kroenke and colleagues [35] found that breast cancer survivors who increased their body mass index by 0.5 to 2 units postdiagnosis were found to have a relative risk of recurrence of 1.40 (95% confidence interval [CI], 1.02–1.92) and those who gained more than 2 body mass index units had a relative risk of 1.53 (95% CI, 1.54–2.34); both groups also experienced significantly higher all-cause mortality. In addition, several studies have reported that increased body weight postdiagnosis negatively impacts QOL [22,32,36]. This accumulating evidence of adverse effects of obesity in cancer survivors, plus evidence indicating that obesity has negative consequences for overall health and physical function, make the pursuit of weight management a priority for cancer survivors [13,22,32], a priority that is substantiated through viable physiologic mechanisms [37] and concern that the health issues of this population are overlaid on the pandemic of overweight and obesity increasing worldwide [37,38].

Despite the documented adverse effects of obesity in cancer survivors, to date only five reported studies have examined weight management in cancer populations, and all were conducted among women with breast cancer. Two of these studies were performed largely on survivors who had completed active treatment, and found that individualized dietary counseling provided by a dietitian was effective in promoting weight loss [39,40]. The more recent study by Djuric and colleagues [40] found that counseling by a dietitian was most effective if combined with a structured Weight Watchers program, which included exercise; weight change at 12 months was +0.85 ± 6 kg versus −8 ± 5.5 kg or −9.4 ± 8.6 kg in the control versus dietitian or dietitian plus Weight Watchers program, respectively. Multiple behavior interventions that use a comprehensive approach to energy balance, and that include both diet and exercise components, have higher likelihood of being more effective than interventions relying on either component alone [41]. In their evaluation of a diet and exercise intervention among early stage breast cancer patients, which was begun during the time of treatment and extended throughout the year following diagnosis, Goodwin and colleagues [42] found that exercise was the strongest predictor of weight loss. These findings were corroborated more recently by the observational study of Herman and colleagues [32]. Given evidence that sarcopenic obesity (gain of adipose tissue at the expense of lean body mass) is a documented side effect of chemotherapy and hormonal therapy [22,43–45], exercise, specifically resistance exercise, may be especially important for cancer survivors because it is considered the cornerstone of treatment for this condition.

Until more is known, guidelines established for weight management in the general population should be applied to cancer survivors, and include not only dietary and exercise components, but also behavior therapy [46]. With research indicating that 71% of cancer survivors are overweight or obese, there is a definite need to develop effective weight management interventions for this needy population [13].

NUTRITION AND DIET

Energy Restriction

Accumulating evidence suggests that weight management should be a priority for cancer survivors [19,20,33]. For most cancer survivors who are overweight, energy-restricted diets are recommended [13,20,21]. Moderate energy deficits of up to 1000 cal/day can be achieved by concomitantly increasing energy expenditure (by exercise) and reducing energy intake [20]. Energy restriction can be achieved by reducing the energy density of the diet by substituting low-energy-density foods (eg, water-rich vegetables, fruits, cooked whole grains, soups) for foods that are higher in calories [47]. This "volumetric approach" enhances satiety and reduces feelings of hunger and deprivation that often serve to undermine energy-restricted diets. An additional strategy is limiting portion sizes of energy-dense foods [47]. The newly issued dietary guidelines for cancer survivors emphasize energy balance and largely endorse dietary recommendations that have been established for the primary prevention of cancer and other chronic diseases [20,38,48].

Balancing Fat, Protein, and Carbohydrate Intake

Protein, carbohydrate, and fat all contribute energy (calories) in the diet, and each of these dietary constituents is available from a wide variety of foods. Making informed choices about foods that provide these macronutrients can ensure variety and nutrient adequacy. In general, the choice of foods and their proportions within an overall diet (dietary pattern) may be more important than absolute amounts [22,38,49]. Given that cancer survivors are at high risk for other chronic diseases, the recommended amounts and type of fat, protein, and carbohydrate to reduce these disease risks also is germane [18,20]. Observational studies of breast cancer survivors (N = 2619) and colorectal cancer survivors (N = 1009) within the Nurse's Health Study cohort suggest that compared with those who reported a Western-type diet (eg, high proportional intakes of meat, refined grains, high-fat dairy products, and desserts), those who reported a prudent diet (eg, high proportional intakes of fruits, vegetables, whole grains, and low-fat dairy products) had significantly better outcomes (ie, improved overall survival and reduced rates of colorectal recurrence and mortality, respectively) [50,51]. Furthermore, cross-sectional data from 714 breast cancer survivors participating in the Health, Eating, Activity and Lifestyle study suggest that postdiagnosis diet quality is significantly associated with mental and physical functioning [52]. Recently, a feasibility study aimed at reducing functional decline among 182 elderly breast and cancer survivors by delivering a multicomponent intervention to increase diet quality and physical activity found evidence of improved physical functioning [53]; this study is currently being followed-up with a full-scale randomized controlled trial entitled Reach-Out to Enhance Wellness (RENEW – CA106919) (N = 641) with results anticipated in 2009.

Fat

To date, roughly 20 reported studies have examined the relationship between fat intake and survival postdiagnosis, with almost all of these studies conducted among breast cancer survivors [17,20,22]. The results tend to be mixed; however, in the few studies that have assessed type of fat there seems to be a consistent finding that high intakes of saturated fat are associated with worse survival [20]. The recently completed Women's Intervention Nutrition Study, a randomized controlled trial that accrued 2437 postmenopausal women within 12 months of breast cancer diagnosis and followed them for roughly 5 years, found a hazards ratio for recurrence of 0.76 (95% CI, 0.60–0.98) among women assigned to the low-fat diet (<15% of energy from fat) compared with those assigned to a nutritionally adequate diet, an effect that was even stronger among participants with estrogen-receptor–negative disease [54]. Although these findings may have been confounded by the 6-lb weight loss observed with the low-fat diet over the course of the study period, these results nonetheless provide support for the US Department of Agriculture recommendations to limit total fat intake to 20% to 35% of energy intake, saturated fat intake to less than 10%, and trans fatty acids to less than 3%, especially in view of the greater risk for cardiovascular disease among survivors [48].

Protein

Relatively few studies have examined associations between protein intake and cancer-specific outcomes, although one study among early stage breast cancer survivors found that increased intakes of red meat, bacon, and liver were associated with increased rates of recurrence [55]. Given these data, and strong evidence that red meat and processed meat are associated with increased primary risk for colorectal cancer, survivors are encouraged to limit their consumption of these foods. Protein intakes of 0.8 g/kg of body weight are recommended with 10% to 35% of energy coming from protein [20,56].

Carbohydrates

Similar to protein, little research has been undertaken with regard to carbohydrates, specifically starches and sugars, and cancer survival. Although fiber is classified as a carbohydrate and its relationship to cancer has been explored extensively, such research has been limited largely to the recurrence of precancerous lesions (eg, colorectal adenomas) more than to survivorship per se [20]. Given that glycemic control is a newly emerging area of interest in relation to cancer, more research is anticipated in this area in the next few years [57]. Given a lack of definitive data, survivors are encouraged to follow dietary guidelines established for the prevention of chronic diseases that endorse intakes of carbohydrates ranging from 45% to 65% of total energy intake and fiber intakes of 14 g/1000 kcal [48]. Carbohydrates should come primarily from nutrient-dense food sources, such as vegetables, whole fruits, and whole grains, low-energy density foods that promote satiety, and weight control, while enhancing nutrient adequacy [20,48]. Refined carbohydrates and sugars are discouraged given their relative lack of nutritional benefit and their contribution to energy intake [20,48].

Vegetables and Fruits

Given high concentrations of various phytochemicals, antioxidants, and fiber, vegetables and fruits have been promoted not only among healthy populations for the prevention of disease but also among cancer survivors [20]. Of a dozen observational studies examining the relationship between intakes of vegetables and fruits (or nutrients indicative of those foods) and risk for cancer recurrence, the evidence has been mixed [20,58,59]. Half of the studies have observed a protective effect of vegetables and fruits or specific items, such as tomato sauce or cruciferae, whereas the remaining studies have found no associations. Results of the Women's Healthy Eating and Living trial, which not only promoted a low-fat, high-fiber diet, but also daily minimum intakes of five vegetable and three fruit servings, and 16 oz of vegetable juice, found no differences in recurrence among 3088 premenopausal and postmenopausal women followed over 7 years [60]. Null findings have been attributed to high baseline vegetables and fruits intakes in both study arms (mean of 7.4 servings per day) or an absence of weight loss, despite a low-energy density diet [61]. Cancer survivors are still encouraged to consume at least five servings of vegetables and fruits per day based on proved cardioprotective effects [20,48].

EXERCISE

Increased attention has focused on the role of exercise training interventions as an adjunct supportive therapy for cancer survivors both during and following the completion of primary therapy. Up to March 2004, 16 independent research investigations had been published examining the role of exercise training interventions in cancer survivors [62–64]. From March 2004 to March 2006, the authors conducted a systematic review that identified nine additional studies for a total of 25 studies of exercise among cancer survivors. To summarize, these studies were conducted predominately in breast cancer survivors testing the effects of either endurance (aerobic) or combined (endurance plus resistance training) exercise training prescribed according to standard exercise prescription guidelines for healthy adults (ie, exercise sessions 3–5 days per week for 20–45 minutes, at a moderate intensity for 2–6 months). Major outcomes of these reports included cardiorespiratory fitness; strength; psychosocial outcomes (eg, QOL, depression, and so forth); and various biochemical outcomes, such as metabolic and sex hormones. The extant literature indicates that exercise training is safe and feasible for cancer survivors following the completion of primary therapy. Moreover, exercise training is associated with a moderately positive effect on cardiorespiratory fitness and QOL. Exercise training also is generally associated with a small positive effect on other outcomes, such as fatigue, anxiety, and depression. Overall, the current literature provides sufficient evidence that exercise is a safe and well-tolerated supportive intervention that physicians can recommend to their patients following the completion of primary therapy [17].

The strength of the evidence is evaluated next in light of studies published within the past year (March 2006–October 2007). A comprehensive review of the literature identified seven new independent studies that examined the effects of an exercise training intervention among cancer survivors that had completed therapy [65–71]. Studies that examined the effects of exercise training in combination with other interventions (eg, dietary interventions) or examined the use of a behavioral-based intervention to promote exercise among cancer survivors were excluded.

These new studies continue to focus predominantly on breast cancer [66–70], with the remaining studies focusing on mixed cancer patients [65,71]. Four studies were randomized controlled trials [66–69], whereas the other three used pre-post designs [65,70,71]. Four studies examined the effects of only aerobic exercise training [66,69–71], two assessed the effects of combined aerobic and resistance training [67,68], and one used only resistance training [65]. The intervention length ranged from 8 to 24 weeks and study end points were various and included exercise capacity (assessed by either a maximal cardiopulmonary exercise test or submaximal treadmill test); muscle strength; and numerous psychosocial outcomes (eg, fatigue, overall QOL, stress, subcomponents of QOL) (see Table 1). Findings from these more recent studies corroborate the prior conclusion that the current literature provides sufficient evidence that exercise is safe and feasible for cancer survivors following the completion of primary therapy and such interventions may be associated with potentially clinically meaningful improvements in exercise capacity and overall QOL. Although not a primary focus of this article, these results also are consistent with the findings of exercise intervention studies conducted during cancer therapy [63]. For example, in the largest study to date, Courneya and colleagues [72] examined the effects of aerobic exercise alone, resistance exercise alone, or usual care on physical fitness, muscle strength, body composition, and indices of QOL and other psychosocial outcomes among 242 operable breast cancer patients initiating adjuvant chemotherapy. Results indicated significant favorable effects of aerobic and resistance exercise training on multiple outcomes (including increased chemotherapy completion rates) compared with usual care without any significant adverse events.

Further strong evidence for the role of exercise for cancer survivors is provided by four landmark studies that examined the association between physical activity and cancer recurrence and overall survival in persons diagnosed with breast [73,74] and colon cancer [75,76]. Results of these studies suggest that survivors who engaged in routine physical activity had a significant disease-free and mortality risk reduction compared with those who were physically inactive. Of note, these findings also include data obtained from women participating in the control arm of the Women's Healthy Eating and Living study, and show that increased physical activity (equivalent of brisk walking for 30 minutes 6 days per week) was associated with a significant reduction in the risk of death among 1490 women with breast cancer, an effect independent of either weight status or vegetables and fruits consumption [74]

Findings from these observational studies have important implications for future exercise interventions focused on cancer survivors. At present, the exercise training studies included in the current article and those reviewed in the prior paper have predominantly focused on the effects of exercise training on exercise capacity and overall QOL [17]. These interventions have included relatively small sample sizes (≤100) with short-term intervention periods (≤6 months) that are prescribed two to three times a week. If exercise training or cancer exercise rehabilitation programs are to become an integral component of multidisciplinary management of cancer survivors, large-scale randomized controlled trials are required that go beyond simply including exercise capacity and QOL outcomes, examine long-term interventions (≥6 months), and prescribe exercise training 3 to 5 days a week, which is consistent with the results of the observational studies and current recommendations of the American Cancer Society, the Centers for Disease Control and Prevention, the American College of Sports Medicine, and the World Health Organization (see Box 2) [38]. Well-designed trials that examine the efficacy of exercise training on biologic mechanisms, derived from preclinical studies, or clinically meaningful intermediate surrogate end points of cancer recurrence or overall survival are urgently required. Findings from studies of this nature provide the necessary evidence to convince policy makers for the inclusion of exercise rehabilitation in cancer management.

SMOKING CESSATION

As noted in the IOM report [18], nearly one third of all cancers are caused by smoking; thus, there is a high likelihood of tobacco use among survivors, especially those who have been diagnosed with smoking-related malignancies (ie, lung, head and neck, cervix, bladder, kidney, pancreas, and myeloid leukemia) [77,78]. Persistent tobacco use postdiagnosis also is associated with poorer outcomes, including increased complications of treatment, progressive disease, second primaries, and increased comorbidity [79,80]. Whereas smoking cessation plays a substantial role in prevention and primary care, it is perhaps even more critical for cancer survivors to quit smoking [81]. Fortunately, many survivors respond to the "teachable moment" that a cancer diagnosis provides [82], and quit rates of approximately 50% are noted among survivors who have smoking-related tumors [12,83]. Unfortunately, data from a recent study suggest that most institutions fail to offer smoking prevention (61%) or cessation (75%) programs to individuals diagnosed with cancer, and many even lack a referral system (42%) [84]. Furthermore, even among survivors who are able to quit, high percentages are unable to remain smoke-free, with approximately one third of smokers continuing to smoke after their cancer diagnosis [12]. Recent data from the National Health Interview Survey also suggest that current smoking rates may be especially high in younger cancer survivors (ages 18–40) than in the general population [85], although subsequent controlled analyses on data with longer follow-up suggest that these differences may not be as discrepant as previously thought [86].

Given evidence that combined interventions that use behavioral counseling along with pharmacotherapy are effective, definitive guidelines exist for providing care as it relates to smoking cessation [18]. The 5-A approach endorsed by the US Preventive Services Task Force provides a concrete framework for health care providers to deliver appropriate care regarding smoking cessation and is a featured element within the IOM report [18,87]. Despite this extant framework, the barriers to long-standing smoking cessation success are substantial and findings from intervention trials have been mixed; the IOM report provides a solid overview of studies conducted up until 2005 and notes the significance of smoking cessation within the survivor population and the numerous barriers that exist [18]. Fortunately, the early trials of Gritz and colleagues [88] and the most recent trial of Emmons and colleagues [89] provide success stories that can guide future treatment, research, and practice. The randomized controlled trial by Emmons and colleagues [89] tested a peer telephone counseling intervention with tailored materials against standardized self-help materials (both with optional nicotine replacement) among 796 currently smoking adult childhood cancer survivors. They found that quit rates were significantly higher in the counseling group compared with the self-help group at both the 8-month (16.8% versus 8.5%; $P < .01$) and 12-month follow-up (15% versus 9%; $P < .01$) [89]. This home-based intervention also was found to be cost-effective. This recent positive trial not only is important for it's contribution to smoking cessation research, but it also paves the way more generally for future health promotion programs by testing innovative strategies that are well-accepted and more readily disseminable to survivor populations who often are hard to reach. As noted in the IOM report [18], opportunities also exist for interventions that incorporate social or familial support as a key element. An ongoing trial that is currently testing the efficacy of such a family-based intervention is entitled "Family-Ties" and results are imminent. As in areas of diet and exercise, more research is necessary to determine interventions that are optimally effective and promote permanent smoking cessation, acknowledging that continued tobacco use may be particularly resistant in cancer survivors. It is also worth noting that smokers may represent a prime population not only for smoking cessation efforts, but also for multiple risk factor interventions, because findings of Butterfield and colleagues [90] suggest that most (63%) cancer survivors who smoke also are likely to engage in at least two to three other unhealthful lifestyle behaviors, such as sedentary behavior, high red meat consumption, and excessive alcohol use.

HEALTH BEHAVIOR CHANGE AND PREFERENCES FOR DELIVERY AMONG CANCER SURVIVORS
Behavior Change Postdiagnosis
Most earlier research suggested that the practice of healthy lifestyle behaviors was higher among cancer survivors than in the general population; however,

recent large-scale studies now indicate that few health behavior differences exist between cancer survivors and healthy populations or noncancer controls [34,85,86]. Two of these studies relied on data collected from survivors of several different cancers and who were nested within a United States sample, which included both cancer cases and controls, yielding data that are less likely to be influenced by responder bias. Analyses by Coups and Ostroff [85] and Bellizzi and colleagues [86] on health behaviors of cancer cases compared with age- and race-matched controls participating in the National Health Initiative Survey-2000 indicate that although cancer survivors are slightly more likely to adhere to physical activity guidelines, for the most part their health behaviors parallel those of the general population: a population marked by inactivity; overweight or obesity; suboptimal fruit, vegetable, and fiber consumption; and high intakes of fat [86]. Similar results were found in another study that exclusively tracked lifestyle behaviors in a cohort of women (N = 2321) with early stage breast cancer [34]. These studies suggest that although many cancer patients report healthful lifestyle changes after diagnosis, these changes may not generalize to all populations of cancer survivors or may be temporary. Given higher rates of comorbidity within this population and evidence that diet, exercise, and tobacco use affect risk for other cancers and other chronic diseases, these recent data support a terrific need for lifestyle interventions that target this vulnerable population.

When is the Best Time to Intervene?

Little data exist as to when cancer survivors may be most receptive to health behavior interventions. An early study of 978 breast and prostate cancer survivors [91] suggests that most (57%) reported a preference for diet, exercise, and smoking cessation information "at diagnosis or soon thereafter" and that a significant decrease ($P = .003$) was noted as time elapsed from diagnosis. Such factors as age and gender also may affect interest and uptake of lifestyle interventions. For example, McBride and colleagues [92] found that interest levels for lifestyle interventions may be sustained over time among women but not in men, because the psychologic impact of disease diminishes significantly with time from diagnosis among males, but not in female survivors.

Timing of interventions also is dependent on the targeted behavior (eg, diet, exercise, and so forth); the channel of delivery (clinic or home-based); treatments received (eg, surgery, radiation, chemotherapy); side effects (fatigue, pain, nausea, and so forth); and desired outcomes (short-term symptom management or overall long-term health). For example, observations from recent studies suggest that interventions involving physical activity may receive better uptake and continued adherence if introduced after primary therapy is complete rather than during active treatment [72,93–95]. Furthermore, such issues as time, transportation, child care, and patients' willingness to undertake new lifestyle behaviors may undermine the success of health promotion efforts and require careful consideration regarding timing, content, delivery channel, and patient selection. Also important is the realization that several strategic iterations may be necessary to create an intervention that not only has proved efficacy, but that also is well-accepted and generalizable to the patient population at large.

Preferred Channels for Delivery

As with intervention timing, there are relatively few studies that have explored patient preferences regarding intervention delivery channel and even fewer that have compared the relative efficacy of different methods. In one study of 307 cancer survivors, Jones and Courneya [96] found that 85% of cancer survivors preferred face-to-face exercise counseling for a one-session class. Other researchers have found that distance and accompanying issues of time and transportation pose significant barriers for in-person programs, especially among older cancer survivors (61% of cancer survivors are 65 years of age or older) [91,97–99]. Such barriers also are present among survivors of more rarely occurring cancers who often have to travel great distances to receive specialized care in appropriate clinical settings (ie, childhood survivors) [100]. In two separate survey studies among breast and prostate cancer survivors [91] and childhood cancer survivors [100], Demark-Wahnefried and colleagues found that distance medicine-based or home-based programs were significantly favored over clinic-based venues. Surprisingly, mailed interventions garnered higher preference scores than computer-based formats among younger cancer survivors. Similarly, Rutten and colleagues [101] reported that cancer survivors were twice as likely to report reliance on print materials as sources of health information rather than the Internet or other media sources. It is currently unknown whether these results are apt to change over time or whether there is a definite hard-set preference for print materials over computer-based venues. Given that cancer is a disease associated with aging and that receptivity for computer-based formats is even lower in older populations, it is safe to say that although web-based programs offer future promise, full penetrance of such programs, especially among the most underserved populations of cancer survivors, is currently questionable [13].

As recently reviewed by Stull and colleagues [102], the preponderance of reported health promotion efforts among cancer survivors have used clinic-based interventions, although increasing numbers of interventions have used hybrid programs that rely on clinic-based sessions with follow-up telephone counseling [13,41]. Although the potential acceptability and reach for home-based interventions is notably greater than for clinic-based programs, to date only five studies have used this approach [53,89,103–105]. Most health promotion interventions among cancer survivors have reported favorable findings, although more research is needed to determine optimal approaches, not only with regard to delivery channel, but also to the previously mentioned areas (ie, timing, pairing of behavioral components, and so forth) [13,102].

SUMMARY

Currently, there is scant evidence regarding the direct impact of postdiagnosis behavioral change on cancer-related progression, recurrence, or survival. Indeed, much more research is necessary, not only to determine proof of concept (ie, that behavior change can make an impact on cancer-specific outcomes and overall health), but also to arrive at interventions that are well-accepted and that reach cancer survivors who are most vulnerable. Research is ongoing and data are beginning to accumulate. In the interim, oncologists should not lose sight of the fact that there exists a significant body of research that shows the benefit of a healthful diet, regular exercise, and smoking cessation for reducing risk for many of the comorbid conditions (ie, other cancers, cardiovascular disease, diabetes, and osteoporosis) and side effects (ie, fatigue and depression) for which cancer survivors are especially prone. Oncology care providers can assist their patients by endorsing existing health guidelines and encouraging their patients to take active roles in pursuing general preventive health strategies.

References

[1] Jemal A, Siegel R, Ward E, et al. Cancer statistics, 2007. CA Cancer J Clin 2007;57: 43–66.

[2] Canadian Cancer Society. Canadian cancer statistics—2007. Available at: http://www.cancer.ca/vgn/images/portal/cit_86751114/36/15/1816216925cw_2007stats_en.pdf. Accessed March 7, 2008.

[3] Rowland J, Mariotto A, Aziz N, et al. Cancer Survivorship—United States. Morbidity and Mortality Weekly Report 2004;53:526–9.

[4] Stricker CT. Endocrine effects of breast cancer treatment. Semin Oncol Nurs 2007;23: 55–70.

[5] Rowland JH, Yancik R. Cancer survivorship: the interface of aging, comorbidity, and quality care. J Natl Cancer Inst 2006;98:504–5.

[6] Nord C, Mykletun A, Thorsen L, et al. Self-reported health and use of health care services in long-term cancer survivors. Int J Cancer 2005;114:307–16.

[7] Eakin EG, Youlden DR, Baade PD, et al. Health status of long-term cancer survivors: results from an Australian population-based sample. Cancer Epidemiol Biomarkers Prev 2006;15:1969–76.

[8] Hooning MJ, Aleman BMP, van Rosmalen AJM, et al. Cause-specific mortality in long-term survivors of breast cancer: a 25-year follow-up study. Int J Radiat Oncol Biol Phys 2006;64: 1081–91.

[9] Hoff AO, Gagel RF. Osteoporosis in breast and prostate cancer survivors. Oncologist 2005;19:651–8.

[10] Chlebowski RT. Bone health in women with early-stage breast cancer. Clin Breast Cancer 2005;5(Suppl):S35–40.

[11] Deimling GT, Sterns S, Wagner LJ, et al. Cancer-related health worries and psychological distress among older adult, long-term cancer survivors. Psychooncology 2006;15(4): 306–20.

[12] Demark-Wahnefried W, Pinto BM, Gritz ER. Promoting health and physical function among cancer survivors: potential for prevention and questions that remain. J Clin Oncol 2006;24(32):5125–31.

[13] Demark-Wahnefried W, Aziz NM, Rowland JH, et al. Riding the crest of the teachable moment: promoting long-term health after the diagnosis of cancer. J Clin Oncol 2005;23: 5814–30.

[14] Carver JR, Shapiro CL, Ng A, et al. American Society of Clinical Oncology clinical evidence review on the ongoing care of adult cancer survivors: cardiac and pulmonary late effects. J Clin Oncol 2007;25:3991–4008.

[15] Baade PD, Fritschi L, Eakin EG. Non-cancer mortality among people diagnosed with cancer (Australia). Cancer Causes Control 2006;17:287–97.

[16] Deimling GT, Sterns S, Bowman KF, et al. The health of older-adult, long-term cancer survivors. Cancer Nurs 2005;28:415–24.

[17] Jones LW, Demark-Wahnefried W, Jones LW, et al. Diet, exercise, and complementary therapies after primary treatment for cancer. Lancet Oncol 2006;7:1017–26.

[18] Hewitt M, Greenfield S, Stovall EL. Institute of Medicine and National Research Council. From cancer patient to cancer survivors: lost in transition. Washington, DC: National Academies Press; 2005.

[19] Jones L, Demark-Wahnefried W. Recommendations for health behavior and wellness following primary treatment for cancer. Washington, DC: National Academies Press; 2007.

[20] Doyle C, Kushi LH, Byers T, et al. Nutrition and physical activity during and after cancer treatment: an American Cancer Society guide for informed choices. CA Cancer J Clin 2006;56:323–53.

[21] Brown JK, Byers T, Doyle C, et al. Nutrition and physical activity during and after cancer treatment: an American Cancer Society guide for informed choices. CA Cancer J Clin 2003;53:268–91.

[22] Rock CL, Demark-Wahnefried W. Nutrition and survival after the diagnosis of breast cancer: a review of the evidence. J Clin Oncol 2002;20:3302–16.

[23] Demark-Wahnefried W. Diet: energy balance and adiposity. In: Brawley O, editor. American Society of Clinical Oncology curriculum: cancer prevention. Alexandria (VA): American Society of Clinical Oncology; 2007. p. 5.1–5.33.

[24] World Health Organization. International Agency for Research in Cancer handbook of cancer prevention. Washington, DC: IARC Press of North America; 2002.

[25] Calle EE, Rodriguez C, Walker-Thurmond K, et al. Overweight, obesity, and mortality from cancer in a prospectively studied cohort of U.S. adults. N Engl J Med 2003;348:1625–38.

[26] Abrahamson PE, Gammon MD, Lund MJ, et al. General and abdominal obesity and survival among young women with breast cancer. Cancer Epidemiol Biomarkers Prev 2006;15:1871–7.

[27] Dignam JJ, Polite BN, Yothers G, et al. Body mass index and outcomes in patients who receive adjuvant chemotherapy for colon cancer. J Natl Cancer Inst 2006;98:1647–54.

[28] Dignam JJ, Wieand K, Johnson KA, et al. Effects of obesity and race on prognosis in lymph node-negative, estrogen receptor-negative breast cancer. Breast Cancer Res Treat 2006;97:245–54.

[29] Reeves KW, Faulkner K, Modugno F, et al. Body mass index and mortality among older breast cancer survivors in the Study of Osteoporotic Fractures. Cancer Epidemiol Biomarkers Prev 2007;16:1468–73.

[30] Tao MH, Shu XO, Ruan ZX, et al. Association of overweight with breast cancer survival. Am J Epidemiol 2006;163:101–7.

[31] Wright ME, Chang S-C, Schatzkin A, et al. Prospective study of adiposity and weight change in relation to prostate cancer incidence and mortality. Cancer 2007;109:675–84.

[32] Herman DR, Ganz PA, Petersen L, et al. Obesity and cardiovascular risk factors in younger breast cancer survivors: the Cancer and Menopause Study (CAMS). Breast Cancer Res Treat 2005;93:13–23.

[33] Chlebowski RT, Aiello E, McTiernan A. Weight loss in breast cancer patient management. J Clin Oncol 2002;20:1128–43.

[34] Caan B, Sternfeld B, Gunderson E, et al. Life After Cancer Epidemiology (LACE) Study: a cohort of early stage breast cancer survivors (United States). Cancer Causes Control 2005;16:545–56.

[35] Kroenke CH, Chen WY, Rosner B, et al. Weight, weight gain, and survival after breast cancer diagnosis. J Clin Oncol 2005;23:1370–8.

[36] Courneya KS, Karvinen KH, Campbell KL, et al. Associations among exercise, body weight, and quality of life in a population-based sample of endometrial cancer survivors. Gynecol Oncol 2005;97:422–30.

[37] Calle EE, Kaaks R. Overweight, obesity and cancer: epidemiological evidence and proposed mechanisms. Nat Rev Cancer 2004;4:579–91.

[38] Work Health Organization. Global strategy on diet, physical activity, and health. Available at: http://www.who.int/dietphysicalactivity. Accessed March 7, 2008.

[39] de Waard F, Ramlau R, Mulders Y, et al. A feasibility study on weight reduction in obese postmenopausal breast cancer patients. Eur J Cancer Prev 1993;2:233–8.

[40] Djuric Z, DiLaura NM, Jenkins I, et al. Combining weight-loss counseling with the weight watchers plan for obese breast cancer survivors. Obes Res 2002;10:657–65.

[41] Agency for Healthcare Research and Quality. Effectiveness of behavioral interventions to modify physical activity behaviors in general populations and cancer patients and survivors. Rockville (MD): U.S. Department of Health and Human Services (AHRQ Publ. No. 04-E027-2); 2004 107–111.

[42] Goodwin P, Esplen MJ, Butler K, et al. Multidisciplinary weight management in locoregional breast cancer: results of a phase II study. Breast Cancer Res Treat 1998;48: 53–64.

[43] Demark-Wahnefried W, Peterson BL, Winer EP, et al. Changes in weight, body composition, and factors influencing energy balance among premenopausal breast cancer patients receiving adjuvant chemotherapy. J Clin Oncol 2001;19:2381–9.

[44] Harvie MN, Howell A, Thatcher N, et al. Energy balance in patients with advanced NSCLC, metastatic melanoma and metastatic breast cancer receiving chemotherapy: a longitudinal study. Br J Cancer 2005;92:673–80.

[45] Smith MR. Changes in body composition during hormonal therapy for prostate cancer. Clin Prostate Cancer 2003;2:18–21.

[46] National Institutes of Health. The practical guide: identification, evaluation, and treatment of overweight and obesity in adults. Am J Clin Nutr 1998;68:899–917.

[47] Rolls BJ, Drewnowski A, Ledikwe JH. Changing the energy density of the diet as a strategy for weight management. J Am Diet Assoc 2005;105:S98–103.

[48] Dietary Guidelines for Americans 2005. Department of Health and Human Services (DHHS), Department of Agriculture (USDA). Available at: http://www.health.gov/dietaryguidelines. Accessed March 7, 2008.

[49] Kennedy ET. Evidence for nutritional benefits in prolonging wellness. Am J Clin Nutr 2006;83:410S–4S.

[50] Kroenke CH, Fung TT, Hu FB, et al. Dietary patterns and survival after breast cancer diagnosis. J Clin Oncol 2005;23:9295–303.

[51] Meyerhardt JA, Niedzwiecki D, Hollis D, et al. Association of dietary patterns with cancer recurrence and survival in patients with stage III colon cancer. JAMA 2007;298: 754–64.

[52] Wayne SJ, Baumgartner K, Baumgartner RN, et al. Diet quality is directly associated with quality of life in breast cancer survivors. Breast Cancer Res Treat 2006;96:227–32.

[53] Demark-Wahnefried W, Clipp EC, Morey MC, et al. Lifestyle intervention development study to improve physical function in older adults with cancer: outcomes from Project LEAD. J Clin Oncol 2006;24:3465–73.

[54] Chlebowski RT, Blackburn GL, Thomson CA, et al. Dietary fat reduction and breast cancer outcome: interim efficacy results from the Women's Intervention Nutrition Study. J Natl Cancer Inst 2006;98:1767–76.

[55] Hebert JR, Hurley TG, Ma Y. The effect of dietary exposures on recurrence and mortality in early stage breast cancer. Breast Cancer Res Treat 1998;51:17–28.

[56] Institute of Medicine. Dietary reference intakes for energy, carbohydrates, fiber, fat, fatty acids, cholesterol, protein, and amino acids. Available at: http://www.iom.edu/CMS/3788/4574.aspx. Accessed March 7, 2008.

[57] Krone CA, Ely JT. Controlling hyperglycemia as an adjunct to cancer therapy. Integr Cancer Ther 2005;4:25–31.

[58] Skuladottir H, Tjoenneland A, Overvad K, et al. Does high intake of fruit and vegetables improve lung cancer survival? Lung Cancer 2006;51:267–73.

[59] Fink BN, Gaudet MM, Britton JA, et al. Fruits, vegetables, and micronutrient intake in relation to breast cancer survival. Breast Cancer Res Treat 2006;98:199–208.

[60] Pierce JP, Natarajan L, Caan BJ, et al. Influence of a diet very high in vegetables, fruit, and fiber and low in fat on prognosis following treatment for breast cancer: the Women's Healthy Eating and Living (WHEL) randomized trial. JAMA 2007;298:289–98.

[61] Agency on Healthcare Research and Quality. Effectiveness of behavioral interventions to modify physical activity behaviors in general populations and cancer patients and survivors. Rockville (MD): US Department of Health and Human Services; 2004. AHRQ Publ. No. 04-E027-2.

[62] McNeely ML, Campbell KL, Rowe BH, et al. Effects of exercise on breast cancer patients and survivors: a systematic review and meta-analysis. CMAJ 2006;175:34–41.

[63] Schmitz KH, Holtzman J, Courneya KS, et al. Controlled physical activity trials in cancer survivors: a systematic review and meta-analysis. Cancer Epidemiol Biomarkers Prev 2005;14:1588–95.

[64] Knols R, Aaronson NK, Uebelhart D, et al. Physical exercise in cancer patients during and after medical treatment: a systematic review of randomized and controlled clinical trials. J Clin Oncol 2005;23:3830–42.

[65] De Backer IC, Van Breda E, Vreugdenhil A, et al. High-intensity strength training improves quality of life in cancer survivors. Acta Oncol 2007. epub ahead of print. PMID: 17851864.

[66] Daley AJ, Crank H, Saxton JM, et al. Randomized trial of exercise therapy in women treated for breast cancer. J Clin Oncol 2007;25:1713–21.

[67] Herrero F, San Juan AF, Fleck SJ, et al. Combined aerobic and resistance training in breast cancer survivors: a randomized, controlled pilot trial. Int J Sports Med 2006;27:573–80.

[68] Milne HM, Wallman KE, Gordon S, et al. Effects of a combined aerobic and resistance exercise program in breast cancer survivors: a randomized controlled trial. Breast Cancer Res Treat 2008;108(2):279–88.

[69] Nikander R, Sievanen H, Ojala K, et al. Effect of a vigorous aerobic regimen on physical performance in breast cancer patients: a randomized controlled pilot trial. Acta Oncol 2007;46:181–6.

[70] Schneider CM, Hsieh CC, Sprod LK, et al. Effects of supervised exercise training on cardiopulmonary function and fatigue in breast cancer survivors during and after treatment. Cancer 2007;110:918–25.

[71] Schneider CM, Hsieh CC, Sprod LK, et al. Exercise training manages cardiopulmonary function and fatigue during and following cancer treatment in male cancer survivors. Integr Cancer Ther 2007;6:235–41.

[72] Courneya KS, Segal RJ, Mackey JR, et al. Effects of aerobic and resistance exercise in breast cancer patients receiving adjuvant chemotherapy: a multicenter randomized controlled trial. J Clin Oncol 2007;25:4396–404.

[73] Holmes MD, Chen WY, Feskanich D, et al. Physical activity and survival after breast cancer diagnosis. JAMA 2005;293:2479–86.

[74] Pierce JP, Stefanick ML, Flatt SW, et al. Greater survival after breast cancer in physically active women with high vegetable-fruit intake regardless of obesity. J Clin Oncol 2007;25:2345–51.

[75] Meyerhardt JA, Giovannucci EL, Holmes MD, et al. Physical activity and survival after colorectal cancer diagnosis. J Clin Oncol 2006;24:3527–34.

[76] Meyerhardt JA, Heseltine D, Niedzwiecki D, et al. Impact of physical activity on cancer recurrence and survival in patients with stage III colon cancer: findings from CALGB 89803. J Clin Oncol 2006;24:3535–41.

[77] International Agency for Research on Cancer. International Agency for Research on Cancer monographs on the evaluation of the carcinogenic risk of chemicals to humans. Lyon (France): International Agency for Research on Cancer Press; 2004.

[78] American Cancer Society. Cancer prevention and early detection. Available at: http://www.cancer.org/docroot/PED/PED_0.asp. Accessed March 7, 2008.

[79] Gritz ER, Dresler C, Sarna L. Smoking, the missing drug interaction in clinical trials: ignoring the obvious. Cancer Epidemiol Biomarkers Prev 2005;14:2287–93.

[80] Lin K, Patel SG, Chu PY, et al. Second primary malignancy of the aerodigestive tract in patients treated for cancer of the oral cavity and larynx. Head Neck 2005;27:1042–8.

[81] Gritz ER, Vidrine DJ, Lazev AB. Smoking cessation in cancer patients: never too late to quit. In: Given B, Given CW, Champion V, et al, editors. Evidence-based interventions in oncology. New York: Springer Publishing Company; 2003. p. 107–40.

[82] McBride CM, Ostroff JS. Teachable moments for promoting smoking cessation: the context of cancer care and survivorship. Cancer Control 2003;10:325–33.

[83] Gritz ER, Fingeret MC, Vidrine DJ, et al. Successes and failures of the teachable moment: smoking cessation in cancer patients. Cancer 2006;106:17–27.

[84] de Moor JS, Puleo E, Butterfield RM, et al. Availability of smoking prevention and cessation services for childhood cancer survivors. Cancer Causes Control 2007;18:423–30.

[85] Coups EJ, Ostroff JS. A population-based estimate of the prevalence of behavioral risk factors among adult cancer survivors and noncancer controls. Prev Med 2005;40:702–11.

[86] Bellizzi KM, Rowland JH, Jeffery DD, et al. Health behaviors of cancer survivors: examining opportunities for cancer control intervention. J Clin Oncol 2005;23:8884–93.

[87] US Preventative Task Force. Counseling to prevent tobacco use and tobacco-related disease: recommendation statement. Available at: http://www.ahrq.gov/clinic/uspstf/uspstbac.htm. Accessed March 7, 2008.

[88] Gritz ER, Carr CR, Rapkin D, et al. Predictors of long-term smoking cessation in head and neck cancer patients. Cancer Epidemiol Biomarkers Prev 1993;2:261–70.

[89] Emmons KM, Puleo E, Park E, et al. Peer-delivered smoking counseling for childhood cancer survivors increases rate of cessation: the partnership for health study. J Clin Oncol 2005;23:6516–23.

[90] Butterfield RM, Park ER, Puleo E, et al. Multiple risk behaviors among smokers in the childhood cancer survivors study cohort. Psychooncology 2004;13:619–29.

[91] Demark-Wahnefried W, Peterson B, McBride C, et al. Current health behaviors and readiness to pursue life-style changes among men and women diagnosed with early stage prostate and breast carcinomas. Cancer 2000;88:674–84.

[92] McBride CM, Clipp E, Peterson BL, et al. Psychological impact of diagnosis and risk reduction among cancer survivors. Psychooncology 2000;9:418–27.

[93] Courneya KS, Mackey JR, Bell GJ, et al. Randomized controlled trial of exercise training in postmenopausal breast cancer survivors: cardiopulmonary and quality of life outcomes. J Clin Oncol 2003;21:1660–8.

[94] Demark-Wahnefried W. Move onward, press forward, and take a deep breath: can lifestyle interventions improve the quality of life of women with breast cancer, and how can we be sure? J Clin Oncol 2007;25:4344–5.

[95] Moadel AB, Shah C, Wylie-Rosett J, et al. Randomized controlled trial of yoga among a multiethnic sample of breast cancer patients: effects on quality of life. J Clin Oncol 2007;25:4387–95.

[96] Jones LW, Courneya KS. Exercise counseling and programming preferences of cancer survivors. Cancer Pract 2002;10:208–15.

[97] Jones LW, Guill B, Keir ST, et al. Exercise interest and preferences among patients diagnosed with primary brain cancer. Support Care in Cancer 2007;15(1):47–55.

[98] Vallance JK, Courneya KS, Jones LW, et al. Exercise preferences among a population-based sample of non-Hodgkin's lymphoma survivors. Eur J Cancer Care (Engl) 2006;15:34–43.

[99] Karvinen KH, Courneya KS, Campbell KL, et al. Exercise preferences of endometrial cancer survivors: a population-based study. Cancer Nurs 2006;29:259–65.

[100] Demark-Wahnefried W, Werner C, Clipp EC, et al. Survivors of childhood cancer and their guardians. Cancer 2005;103:2171–80.

[101] Rutten LJ, Arora NK, Bakos AD, et al. Information needs and sources of information among cancer patients: a systematic review of research (1980–2003). Patient Educ Couns 2005;57:250–61.

[102] Stull VB, Snyder DC, Demark-Wahnefried W. Lifestyle interventions in cancer survivors: designing programs that meet the needs of this vulnerable and growing population. J Nutr 2007;137:243S–8S.

[103] Demark-Wahnefried W, Clipp EC, Lipkus IM, et al. Main outcomes of the FRESH START trial: a sequentially tailored, diet and exercise mailed print intervention among breast and prostate cancer survivors. J Clin Oncol 2007;25:2709–18.

[104] Vallance JKH, Courneya KS, Plotnikoff RC, et al. Randomized controlled trial of the effects of print materials and step pedometers on physical activity and quality of life in breast cancer survivors. J Clin Oncol 2007;25:2352–9.

[105] Wilson RW, Jacobsen PB, Fields KK. Pilot study of a home-based aerobic exercise program for sedentary cancer survivors treated with hematopoietic stem cell transplantation. Bone Marrow Transplant 2005;35:721–7.

Integrative Oncology: Complementary Therapies for Cancer Survivors

Kathleen Wesa, MD, Jyothirmai Gubili, MS*,
Barrie Cassileth, MS, PhD

Integrative Medicine Service, Memorial Sloan-Kettering Cancer Center, 1429 First Avenue
(at 74th Street), New York, NY 10021, USA

Complementary and alternative therapies are being increasingly sought by cancer patients for control of cancer and treatment-related symptoms. Even though these therapies are grouped under a common heading, the differences between the two are profound. Alternative therapies are expensive, frequently harmful, and can interact with chemotherapy drugs and other medications. In contrast, complementary therapies, such as acupuncture, meditation, music, and massage, are noninvasive techniques applied to control symptoms commonly experienced by cancer patients. These therapies are used as adjuncts to standard treatments to improve quality of life. Patients and physicians should be aware of this important distinction.

Cancer survivors experience a wide range of symptoms during and following completion of treatment, and some of these symptoms may persist for years or even decades. While pharmacologic treatments relieve many symptoms, they too may produce difficult side effects. Complementary therapies are noninvasive, inexpensive, and useful in controlling symptoms and improving quality of life, and they may be accessed by patients themselves. The Appendix at the end of this article lists reliable sources of information on complementary therapies.

Complementary therapies are used as adjuncts to mainstream medical care. They are to be distinguished from "alternative" therapies, which are unproven or disproved methods often promoted as viable treatment options. Alternative therapies may be harmful and can jeopardize patients' lives, especially when patients delay needed care. The terms "integrative medicine" or "integrative oncology" are increasingly used worldwide to differentiate between unproven or unsafe practices and today's evidence-based complementary therapies and the study of botanicals. The change in terminology has been accompanied by the application and insistence on rigorous evidence, as indicated by the following examples.

*Corresponding author. E-mail address: gubilij@mskcc.org (J. Gubili).

0889-8588/08/$ – see front matter
doi:10.1016/j.hoc.2008.02.002

The Society for Integrative Oncology (SIO), an international nonprofit organization established to encourage scientific evaluation, dissemination of evidence-based information, and appropriate clinical integration of complementary therapies was established in 2004, and its journal, the JSIO, followed. In 2007, Integrative Oncology Practice Guidelines were published [1], as were practice guidelines for lung cancer by the American College of Chest Physicians [2].

The National Institutes of Health's (NIH) Center for Complementary and Alternative Medicine classifies popular and culturally historic medical approaches into five categories:

Manipulative and body-based practices, including chiropractic or osteopathic manipulation or massage therapy;

Whole medical systems, such as traditional Chinese medicine from China or Ayurveda from India;

Mind-body medicine, which includes meditation, prayer, and creative outlets such as art, music, and dance;

Biologically-based practices, such as herbs, foods, and other substances found in nature, as well as dietary supplements; and

Energy medicine, the manipulation of purported energy fields.

With the likely exception of energy medicine, these categories include potentially useful, evidence-based therapies that can serve well as adjuncts to mainstream cancer care. They are relevant to patient care throughout treatment, and especially important to survivors whose emotional and physical symptoms continue beyond completion of treatment. These evidence-based integrative modalities are discussed in further detail below. They include:

Massage therapies from ancient traditions

Acupuncture from traditional Chinese medicine

Mind-body practices, such as meditation, yoga, hypnosis, and music therapy

Fitness, including exercise and nutritional guidance

Botanical agents from the NIH "Biologically Based Practices" category.

MASSAGE THERAPY

Massage therapy is the application of pressure on muscle and connective tissue to reduce pain, relieve tension and anxiety, and promote relaxation. Therapeutic massage ranges from very light touch to deeper tissue pressure, depending on the patient's clinical status. Deep tissue massage should be reserved for patients with normal blood counts but should not occur immediately after surgery. Foot massage (reflexology) is highly valued by patients, and may be preferable for patients who are frail or uncomfortable with body massage.

Massage therapy is used adjunctively in the treatment of many illnesses. It can decrease pain, fatigue, stress and anxiety [3–5], nausea [6], and depression by approximately 50% on average. Such decreases in symptoms have been found even for patients with a very high baseline score, and may provide symptom relief for 48 hours or more [7]. Reflexology or foot massage relieves anxiety and pain when administered by a trained therapist or by the patient's caregiver [8]. Foot massage can be taught to family members, offering an additional and cost-effective treatment benefit for application in patients' homes.

Massage therapy possesses a very favorable risk-benefit ratio, with a low likelihood of harmful side effects. It is an important complementary therapy for symptom management for survivors, as well as patients in all stages of cancer treatment and management.

ACUPUNCTURE

Acupuncture, an important component of traditional Chinese medicine, has been used for millennia. Most other Asian medical traditions, such as those in Japan, Korea, and Tibet, also included and continue to use acupuncture. The theory underlying acupuncture is that the body contains vertical energy channels, called meridians, through which "qi" (pronounced "chee") or energy flows. Disease is said to occur when the meridians become blocked, preventing the free flow of qi. Acupuncture needles or physical pressure on acupuncture points was believed to unblock the meridians and stimulate the normal, smooth flow of qi, thereby enabling the return to health.

Although recent studies show that meridians correspond to connective tissue planes, there is no verifiable anatomic foundation for the ancient and admirable meridian and qi concept. Modern research, however, does verify acupuncture's specific physiologic effects. It is a well-documented means of reducing cancer and cancer-treatment related symptoms. Multiple well designed studies support the use of acupuncture for nausea [9,10], and even stimulation of the relevant acupuncture point on the wrist with acupressure wrist bands relieves acute nausea [11–14]; it is less effective against prolonged nausea [13]. Electro-acupuncture [15] also controls pain [16–18].

Xerostomia, or extreme dry mouth following head and neck radiation therapy, may be improved with acupuncture treatment, even for patients who have suffered xerostomia for years [19]. Acupuncture also may speed recovery following abdominal surgery; 92% of those receiving acupuncture versus 46% of control subjects recovered bowel function at 72 hours following an operation [20]. Vasomotor symptoms of hot flashes and depression also decrease following acupuncture [21,22]. Weekly electroacupuncture for a 12-week period decreased hot flashes by more than 50% at 6 months after treatment follow-up. Patients also report that their fatigue was decreased by acupuncture.

MIND-BODY THERAPIES

Various mind-body techniques, such as meditation, hypnosis, relaxation and cognitive-behavioral therapies, biofeedback, and guided imagery are increasingly popular and available as part of mainstream medical care. According to a meta-analysis of 116 studies, mind-body practices decrease anxiety, depression, and mood disturbance in cancer patients, and improve coping skills [23]. An important aspect of the mind-body therapies is that regular practice is required for full benefit. Incorporating these techniques into the daily routine helps to ensure ongoing benefit for cancer survivors.

A 2003 survey of United States adults showed that 12% of respondents had used deep breathing exercises and 8% had used meditation in the previous 12-month period [24]. A substantial number of people practice yoga.

Yoga

Yoga is a 5,000-year-old exercise regimen developed in India. Research documents its value in improving physical fitness and decreasing respiratory rate and blood pressure, and yoga is often included in integrative management for heart disease, asthma, and arthritis, as well as cancer.

Yoga also involves focused breath awareness combined with an inward mental focus, which facilitates the mind-body connection. This combination of breath awareness, mental focus, and physical movement assists in parasympathetic nervous system predominance, which dampens the stress response. One study of lymphoma patients used a Tibetan yoga sequence involving mindfulness techniques, controlled breathing, visualization, and low-impact physical yoga postures. Significantly lower sleep disturbance scores, better subjective sleep quality, decreased sleep latency, longer sleep duration, and decreased use of sleeping medication in the yoga group compared with wait-list controls were found [25].

Four recent studies of breast cancer patients showed significant quality of life benefits following weekly yoga classes over an 8- to 12-week period. Improvements were observed in emotional well being and distressed mood [26–29]. Of the participants, 69% attended at least half of the classes, suggesting that even intermittent attendance at yoga sessions can provide significant emotional benefit [29]. A study of women undergoing radiotherapy for breast cancer showed a significant decrease in depression and anxiety when compared with controls [26].

Increased physical and emotional benefits are also reported for breast cancer survivors an average of 56 months following diagnosis in a 7-week study [28]. Yoga is beneficial even for those with metastatic disease, according to a study of gentle yoga postures, breathing exercises, meditation, didactic presentations, and group interchange in women with metastatic breast cancer. A significant decrease in pain and fatigue was found following each of eight weekly sessions [27].

Meditation

There are numerous meditation techniques with various practitioners applying their own descriptive terminology and emphases. Regardless of its name, meditation involves inducing a calm state of mind by oneself or with the help of another. Mindfulness based stress reduction (MBSR), for example, combines mindfulness meditation with yoga poses to help patients cope with stress, pain, and illness by promoting moment-to-moment awareness. The curriculum consists of 45-minute sessions 6 days per week over an 8-week period. Daily practice alternates between mindfulness meditation, breath awareness, and yoga poses. The training program culminates with a 6-hour silent session combining the different mindfulness techniques learned over the course. MBSR has been shown consistently to decrease stress levels and blood pressure, and to enhance mood and immune function in cancer patients [30–34].

A study of 63 cancer outpatients examined the effects of an 8-week MBSR program on sleep, mood, stress, and fatigue. Overall sleep disturbance was significantly reduced ($P < .001$) and participants reported that their sleep quality had improved ($P = .001$). Significant reductions also occurred for stress ($P < .001$), mood disturbance ($P = .001$), and fatigue ($P < .001$) [35]. Many hospitals and universities provide classes in MBSR, educational books are available, and retreats are offered for those who want a more intensive MBSR experience.

Less intense meditation practices include breath awareness practices, where the attention is focused on the breath and the sensation of breathing at the level of the nostrils as well as the abdominal region; loving kindness meditations, where loving thoughts are focused toward other persons; mantra meditation, where a word or phrase is mentally repeated silently as a method of focusing the mind; and contemplative meditation, where the meaning of a word or phrase is contemplated in the effort of further understanding its meaning. The different meditation techniques produce similar physiologic response, with the resulting benefit of stress reduction and improved mood.

Hypnosis

Hypnosis is a state of focused attention or altered consciousness between wakefulness and sleep in which distractions are blocked, allowing a person to concentrate intently on a particular subject, memory, sensation, or problem. In essence, it is a deeper form of meditation. During the hypnotic state, a suggestion is supplanted, which is geared to affect the desired results. Hypnosis can be self-administered or performed by a trained therapist. It has been studied extensively and found effective for a wide range of symptoms, including acute and chronic pain, panic, phobias, and preoperative symptom management.

A recent randomized clinical trial compared a 15-minute presurgery hypnosis session conducted by a psychologist with a nondirective empathic listening session on 200 persons undergoing excisional breast biopsy or lumpectomy. The group receiving the preoperative hypnosis experienced significantly less pain, nausea, fatigue, discomfort, and emotional upset at discharge when compared with the control group. In addition, the subjects who received hypnosis had faster recovery, earlier discharge, and institutional cost savings [36].

Thirty subjects scheduled for an interventional radiology procedure were randomized to hypnosis or standard care. Patients in the hypnosis group reported less pain compared with those in the standard care group [37]. This principal can be generalized to survivors while they await a similarly stressful experience, such as a scan to determine clinical status. Hypnosis can also control nausea and vomiting. A randomized controlled trial of 50 breast surgery subjects taught presurgical hypnosis showed that subjects in the hypnosis group experienced 29% less vomiting compared with standard-care controls [38].

Hypnosis can also be effective in children. Fifty-four pediatric cancer patients were randomly assigned to hypnosis, nonhypnotic distraction and relaxation, or attention control. Children in the hypnosis group reported the greatest reduction in anticipatory and after chemotherapy nausea and vomiting [39].

MUSIC THERAPY

Music is a powerful tool that can evoke latent emotions, induce a range of emotional states, and enhance communication. Music therapy is provided by trained musicians who hold professional degrees in music therapy. They manage psychosocial issues faced by patients and family members with music rather than words. It offers creative, lyrical, and symbolic means to address existential and spiritual needs, as well as communication and psychosocial problems. Many major institutions offer music therapy programs. Controlled trials indicate that music therapy produces emotional and physiologic benefits by reducing anxiety, stress, depression, and pain. It is also effective against laboratory-induced pain among cancer patients [40] and among cancer patients with chronic pain [41]. In what was possibly the largest trial of its type, 500 surgical subjects were randomized to control, recorded music, jaw relaxation, or a music and jaw relaxation combination. Music led to significant decreases in both pain intensity and related distress associated with pain [42].

Music can also help reduce depression. In a randomized controlled trial of cancer subjects undergoing autologous stem cell transplantation, anxiety, depression, and total mood disturbance scores were significantly lower in the music therapy group when compared with standard-care controls [43].

FITNESS

The importance of diet, nutrition, and physical fitness on survivorship and quality of life issues must not be overlooked. Research has shown that when provided with sequentially tailored information on how to improve one's diet through increasing fruit and vegetable consumption, reducing total saturated fat intake, and increasing physical activity, cancer survivors are able to significantly improve their lifestyle behaviors [44,45]. While no diet has been shown to treat cancer, eating a healthy diet has been associated with improvement in cardiovascular disease, diabetes, and obesity, all of which improve survival.

In the past year there have been numerous studies demonstrating the beneficial effects of exercise and physical fitness. One study of 242 breast cancer subjects receiving adjuvant chemotherapy demonstrated that both aerobic and resistance exercise significantly improved self-esteem, physical fitness, body composition, and chemotherapy completion rate when compared with usual care [46]. Changes in cancer-specific quality of life, as well as symptoms of fatigue, depression, and anxiety, favored the exercise groups over usual care, but did not reach statistical significance. A British study showed that aerobic exercise or body conditioning showed significant improvements in quality of life measurements of social and family well being, functional well being, and psychologic benefits when compared with usual care [47].

Although both resistance exercise and aerobic exercise are beneficial, one study examined the results of aerobic exercise, resistance exercise, or usual care in women undergoing adjuvant chemotherapy. The results showed that weight-bearing aerobic exercise attenuates declines in bone mineral density and that both the aerobic and resistance exercise improved aerobic capacity and muscle strength at a time when women generally show marked declines in their functional ability [48]. Thus exercise, and specifically aerobic weight-bearing exercise, may prevent or at least minimize bone loss observed during chemotherapy and may prevent or delay the long-term effects of osteoporosis. Adequate calcium and Vitamin D supplementation is also an important factor for minimizing bone density decline in cancer survivors [49].

HERBS AND BOTANICALS

Plants have been used as medicine since ancient times by all cultures. Medicinal herbal agents, also termed phytomedicinals, are made from the whole plant or its leaves, stems, flowers, seeds, or roots. Herbal supplements may consist of a single herb or a combination of several herbs, as is typical of traditional Chinese medicine and Ayurvedic medicine from India.

Since 1994, botanicals have been regulated under the Dietary Supplement Health and Education Act. Botanicals are considered as dietary supplements and are not regulated by the Food and Drug Administration (FDA). Many dietary supplements, including botanical preparations, are produced with minimal, if any quality control. The FDA does not review botanicals for their safety or effectiveness, requiring manufacturers only to state that their product is not intended to diagnose, treat, cure, or prevent any disease. Claims regarding the product's effect on structure, function, or of general well being and benefits related to nutrient-deficiencies are permitted. While the FDA does not approve the use of botanicals, they may ban these agents if they are proven unsafe for human consumption.

Cancer patients and survivors tend to use herbal supplements to alleviate symptoms, although a majority expect the botanical agent to suppress tumor growth [50,51]. The public typically considers herbs and other botanicals as "natural" and "safe," compared with invasive treatments with serious side effects.

Although some botanicals have beneficial effects, studies indicate that the misuse of herbs can be detrimental. For example, herbs such as ginger, ginseng, garlic, and ginkgo have antiplatelet effects that may cause postoperative hemorrhage [52], and mildly estrogenic botanicals, such as red clover and soy, may stimulate the growth of hormonal sensitive cancers [53,54]. Other botanicals may interfere with prescription medications through multiple mechanisms, including the induction or inhibition of metabolic enzymes, resulting in altered serum levels.

The use of antioxidant agents during chemotherapy and radiotherapy is highly controversial, as the evidence regarding their safety is conflicting. Until high quality research definitively shows lack of harm, it is strongly recommended that cancer patients avoid botanical and other supplement use during receipt of chemotherapy or radiotherapy, before surgery, and when on prescription medications.

An additional concern with botanical agents is contamination by pesticides, heavy metals, microbials, and extraneous material. This may especially be of concern for imported botanical products or products grown in contaminated soil. Quality control is an additional issue, as the botanical content actually present may vary greatly across product lots. It is important to purchase products from reputable manufacturers and suppliers, with quality control effort indicated on the label, to minimize product variability and maximize product quality.

Herbal supplements are not viable substitutes for mainstream cancer treatment. Cancer patients and survivors on prescription pharmaceuticals should approach herbal products with caution, as herb-drug interactions are not uncommon. The Memorial Sloan-Kettering Cancer Center's "About Herbs" Web site is an excellent resource for both physicians and patients, containing continually updated monographs on over 232 botanical and nutritional supplements (see the Appendix at the end of this article) [52].

SUMMARY

Complementary therapies are used for symptom management, not for tumor treatment per se. These therapies control side effects from the cancer, as well as long-term toxicities resulting from chemotherapy, radiation, and surgery. Complementary therapies also offer patients the opportunity to select adjunctive treatments suited to their needs and to participate actively in their own recovery and survivorship. Public interest in these therapies has resulted in a multibillion dollar business in the United States and in other developed countries.

Although many complementary therapies have been practiced over time as components of traditional medical systems worldwide, rigorous scientific research has been applied primarily in the past decade. This research has produced evidence that acupuncture, massage therapy, music, and mind-body therapies effectively and safely reduce physical and emotional symptoms. These therapies provide a favorable risk-benefit ratio and permit cancer survivors to help manage their own care. Botanical and other nutritional supplements may produce unintended interactions with pharmaceuticals or exert undesirable effects. Cancer survivors and their physicians should be alert to these possibilities.

APPENDIX: RELIABLE SOURCES OF INFORMATION ON COMPLEMENTARY THERAPIES

Medline Plus: http://www.nlm.nih.gov/medlineplus/druginformation.html

British Medical Journal: http://www.biomedcentral.com/bmccomplemental ternmed/

Memorial Sloan-Kettering Cancer Center: http://www.mskcc.org/aboutherbs

National Center for Complementary and Alternative Medicine: http://nccam.nih.gov

American Cancer Society: http://www.cancer.org/docroot/ETO/ETO_5.asp?sitearea=ETO

NIH Office of Dietary Supplements: http://dietary-supplements.info.nih.gov

United States Pharmacopeia: http://www.usp.org/dietarySupplements

References

[1] Deng GE, Cassileth BR, Cohen L, et al. Integrative oncology practice guidelines. J Soc Integr Oncol 2007;5(2):65–84.

[2] Cassileth BR, Deng GE, Gomez JE, et al. Complementary therapies and integrative oncology in lung cancer: ACCP evidence-based clinical practice guidelines (2nd edition). Chest 2007;132(Suppl 3):340S–54S.

[3] Field T, Hernandez-Reif M, Diego M, et al. Cortisol decreases and serotonin and dopamine increase following massage therapy. Int J Neurosci 2005;115(10):1397–413.

[4] Goodfellow LM. The effects of therapeutic back massage on psychophysiologic variables and immune function in spouses of patients with cancer. Nurs Res 2003;52(5):318–28.

[5] Hernandez-Reif M, Ironson G, Field T, et al. Breast cancer patients have improved immune and neuroendocrine functions following massage therapy. J Psychosom Res 2004;57(1):45–52.

[6] Billhult A, Bergbom I, Stener-Victorin E. Massage relieves nausea in women with breast cancer who are undergoing chemotherapy. J Altern Complement Med 2007;13(1):53–7.

[7] Cassileth BR, Vickers AJ. Massage therapy for symptom control: outcome study at a major cancer center. J Pain Symptom Manage 2004;28(3):244–9.

[8] Stephenson NL, Swanson M, Dalton J, et al. Partner-delivered reflexology: effects on cancer pain and anxiety. Oncol Nurs Forum 2007;34(1):127–32.

[9] Gan TJ, Jiao KR, Zenn M, et al. A randomized controlled comparison of electro-acupoint stimulation or ondansetron versus placebo for the prevention of postoperative nausea and vomiting. Anesth Analg 2004;99(4):1070–5, table of contents.

[10] Shen J, Wenger N, Glaspy J, et al. Electroacupuncture for control of myeloablative chemotherapy-induced emesis: A randomized controlled trial. JAMA 2000;284(21):2755–61.

[11] Dibble SL, Chapman J, Mack KA, et al. Acupressure for nausea: results of a pilot study. Oncol Nurs Forum 2000;27(1):41–7.

[12] Roscoe JA, Jean-Pierre P, Morrow GR, et al. Exploratory analysis of the usefulness of acupressure bands when severe chemotherapy-related nausea is expected. J Soc Integr Oncol 2006;4(1):16–20.

[13] Roscoe JA, Matteson SE, Morrow GR, et al. Acustimulation wrist bands are not effective for the control of chemotherapy-induced nausea in women with breast cancer. J Pain Symptom Manage 2005;29(4):376–84.

[14] Roscoe JA, Morrow GR, Hickok JT, et al. The efficacy of acupressure and acustimulation wrist bands for the relief of chemotherapy-induced nausea and vomiting. A University of Rochester Cancer Center Community Clinical Oncology Program multicenter study. J Pain Symptom Manage 2003;26(2):731–42.

[15] Minton O, Higginson IJ. Electroacupuncture as an adjunctive treatment to control neuropathic pain in patients with cancer. J Pain Symptom Manage 2007;33(2):115–7.

[16] Alimi D, Rubino C, Pichard-Leandri E, et al. Analgesic effect of auricular acupuncture for cancer pain: a randomized, blinded, controlled trial. J Clin Oncol 2003;21(22):4120–6.

[17] Dang W, Yang J. Clinical study on acupuncture treatment of stomach carcinoma pain. J Tradit Chin Med 1998;18(1):31–8.

[18] Zhang T, Ma SL, Xie GR, et al. Clinical research on nourishing yin and unblocking meridians recipe combined with opioid analgesics in cancer pain management. Chin J Integr Med 2006;12(3):180–4.

[19] Blom M, Dawidson I, Fernberg JO, et al. Acupuncture treatment of patients with radiation-induced xerostomia. Eur J Cancer B Oral Oncol 1996;32B(3):182–90.

[20] Wan Q. Auricular-plaster therapy plus acupuncture at zusanli for postoperative recovery of intestinal function. J Tradit Chin Med 2000;20(2):134–5.

[21] Nedstrand E, Wijma K, Wyon Y, et al. Vasomotor symptoms decrease in women with breast cancer randomized to treatment with applied relaxation or electro-acupuncture: a preliminary study. Climacteric 2005;8(3):243–50.

[22] Nedstrand E, Wyon Y, Hammar M, et al. Psychological well-being improves in women with breast cancer after treatment with applied relaxation or electro-acupuncture for vasomotor symptom. J Psychosom Obstet Gynaecol 2006;27(4):193–9.

[23] Devine EC, Westlake SK. The effects of psychoeducational care provided to adults with cancer: meta-analysis of 116 studies. Oncol Nurs Forum 1995;22(9):1369–81.

[24] Barnes PM, Powell-Griner E, McFann K, et al. Complementary and alternative medicine use among adults: United States, 2002. Adv Data 2004;343:1–19.

[25] Cohen L, Warneke C, Fouladi RT, et al. Psychological adjustment and sleep quality in a randomized trial of the effects of a Tibetan yoga intervention in patients with lymphoma. Cancer 2004;100(10):2253–60.

[26] Banerjee B, Vadiraj HS, Ram A, et al. Effects of an integrated yoga program in modulating psychological stress and radiation-induced genotoxic stress in breast cancer patients undergoing radiotherapy. Integr Cancer Ther 2007;6(3):242–50.

[27] Carson JW, Carson KM, Porter LS, et al. Yoga for women with metastatic breast cancer: results from a pilot study. J Pain Symptom Manage 2007;33(3):331–41.

[28] Culos-Reed SN, Carlson LE, Daroux LM, et al. A pilot study of yoga for breast cancer survivors: physical and psychological benefits. Psychooncology 2006;15(10):891–7.

[29] Moadel AB, Shah C, Wylie-Rosett J, et al. Randomized controlled trial of yoga among a multiethnic sample of breast cancer patients: effects on quality of life. J Clin Oncol 2007;25(28):4344–5.

[30] Carlson LE, Speca M, Patel KD, et al. Mindfulness-based stress reduction in relation to quality of life, mood, symptoms of stress, and immune parameters in breast and prostate cancer outpatients. Psychosom Med 2003;65(4):571–81.

[31] Carlson LE, Speca M, Patel KD, et al. Mindfulness-based stress reduction in relation to quality of life, mood, symptoms of stress and levels of cortisol, dehydroepiandrosterone sulfate (DHEAS) and melatonin in breast and prostate cancer outpatients. Psychoneuroendocrinology 2004;29(4):448–74.

[32] Carlson LE, Ursuliak Z, Goodey E, et al. The effects of a mindfulness meditation-based stress reduction program on mood and symptoms of stress in cancer outpatients: 6-month follow-up. Support Care Cancer 2001;9(2):112–23.

[33] Smith JE, Richardson J, Hoffman C, et al. Mindfulness-Based Stress Reduction as supportive therapy in cancer care: systematic review. J Adv Nurs 2005;52(3):315–27.

[34] Carlson LE, Speca M, Patel KD, et al. One year pre-post intervention follow-up of psychological, immune, endocrine and blood pressure outcomes of mindfulness-based stress reduction (MBSR) in breast and prostate cancer outpatients. Brain Behav Immun 2007;21(8):1038–49.

[35] Carlson LE, Garland SN. Impact of mindfulness-based stress reduction (MBSR) on sleep, mood, stress and fatigue symptoms in cancer outpatients. Int J Behav Med 2005;12(4):278–85.

[36] Montgomery GH, Bovbjerg DH, Schnur JB, et al. A randomized clinical trial of a brief hypnosis intervention to control side effects in breast surgery patients. J Natl Cancer Inst 2007;99(17):1304–12.
[37] Lang EV, Joyce JS, Spiegel D, et al. Self-hypnotic relaxation during interventional radiological procedures: effects on pain perception and intravenous drug use. Int J Clin Exp Hypn 1996;44(2):106–19.
[38] Enqvist B, Bjorklund C, Engman M, et al. Preoperative hypnosis reduces postoperative vomiting after surgery of the breasts. A prospective, randomized and blinded study. Acta Anaesthesiol Scand 1997;41(8):1028–32.
[39] Zeltzer LK, Dolgin MJ, LeBaron S, et al. A randomized, controlled study of behavioral intervention for chemotherapy distress in children with cancer. Pediatrics 1991;88(1):34–42.
[40] Beck SL. The therapeutic use of music for cancer-related pain. Oncol Nurs Forum 1991;18(8):1327–37.
[41] Zimmerman L, Pozehl B, Duncan K, et al. Effects of music in patients who had chronic cancer pain. West J Nurs Res 1989;11(3):298–309.
[42] Good M, Stanton-Hicks M, Grass JA, et al. Relaxation and music to reduce postsurgical pain. J Adv Nurs 2001;33(2):208–15.
[43] Cassileth BR, Vickers AJ, Magill LA. Music therapy for mood disturbance during hospitalization for autologous stem cell transplantation: a randomized controlled trial. Cancer 2003;98(12):2723–9.
[44] Demark-Wahnefried W, Clipp EC, Lipkus IM, et al. Main outcomes of the FRESH START trial: a sequentially tailored, diet and exercise mailed print intervention among breast and prostate cancer survivors. J Clin Oncol 2007;25(19):2709–18.
[45] Vallance JK, Courneya KS, Plotnikoff RC, et al. Randomized controlled trial of the effects of print materials and step pedometers on physical activity and quality of life in breast cancer survivors. J Clin Oncol 2007;25(17):2352–9.
[46] Courneya KS, Segal RJ, Mackey JR, et al. Effects of aerobic and resistance exercise in breast cancer patients receiving adjuvant chemotherapy: a multicenter randomized controlled trial. J Clin Oncol 2007;25(28):4396–404.
[47] Daley AJ, Crank H, Saxton JM, et al. Randomized trial of exercise therapy in women treated for breast cancer. J Clin Oncol 2007;25(13):1713–21.
[48] Schwartz AL, Winters-Stone K, Gallucci B. Exercise effects on bone mineral density in women with breast cancer receiving adjuvant chemotherapy. Oncol Nurs Forum 2007;34(3):627–33.
[49] Ryan CW, Huo D, Stallings JW, et al. Lifestyle factors and duration of androgen deprivation affect bone mineral density of patients with prostate cancer during first year of therapy. Urology 2007;70(1):122–6.
[50] Hyodo I, Amano N, Eguchi K, et al. Nationwide survey on complementary and alternative medicine in cancer patients in Japan. J Clin Oncol 2005;23(12):2645–54.
[51] Molassiotis A, Fernadez-Ortega P, Pud D, et al. Use of complementary and alternative medicine in cancer patients: a European survey. Ann Oncol 2005;16(4):655–63.
[52] Deng G, Cassileth BR. To what extent do cancer patients use complementary and alternative medicine? Nat Clin Pract Oncol 2005;2(10):496–7.
[53] Beck V, Unterrieder E, Krenn L, et al. Comparison of hormonal activity (estrogen, androgen and progestin) of standardized plant extracts for large scale use in hormone replacement therapy. J Steroid Biochem Mol Biol 2003;84(2–3):259–68.
[54] Hsieh CY, Santell RC, Haslam SZ, et al. Estrogenic effects of genistein on the growth of estrogen receptor-positive human breast cancer (MCF-7) cells in vitro and in vivo. Cancer Res 1998;58(17):3833–8.

Cancer Survivorship: Advocacy Organizations and Support Systems

Susan Leigh, BSN, RN

5050 East Golder Ranch Road, Tucson, AZ 85739, USA

Advocacy is simply being a voice for the vulnerable—PJ Haylock, RN, personal communication, 2007

When oncology evolved into a specialized field of medicine more than 4 decades ago, the primary goals of most cancer treatment was to extend patients' lives and to offer occasional hope for a cure. Physicians were seen as the principal and solitary advocate for patients, and information regarding cancer diagnosis, treatment, and side effects was delivered or screened by a doctor. Patient education materials were scarce, formalized support systems were nonexistent, and the future was difficult to define.

Fast-forward to 2007, and cancer care has entered a new era. In the intervening decades, handwritten notes developed into Internet searches and downloaded articles. Mimeographed newsletters became high-quality patient education publications. Advocacy expanded from sole physician guidance to models of self, organizational, and public policy advocacy. Moreover, quality cancer care began its evolution from simple medical treatment that focused on the disease to a more integrative approach that included psychologic, social, and spiritual care. The Internet/information age has literally exploded into the lives of health care providers and cancer survivors such that it is difficult to remain abreast of the latest developments.

Meanwhile, our medical successes have expanded the need for more intricate and continued care of cancer survivors. Therapies have become complicated, and patients who have metastatic disease live longer with more treatment options. Long-term survivors are often cured of their original disease, yet develop secondary malignancies or suffer other consequences of earlier treatments. Consequently, the demand for increased resources for cancer survivors reflects the increased need brought about by treatment success, including information on the long-term complications of cancer and its therapy. This article provides examples of advocacy organizations and support systems that offer guidance to providers and patients throughout the continuum of cancer care and into longer-term survival. By no means is this intended as a comprehensive list, but

E-mail address: sleigh@mindspring.com

0889-8588/08/$ – see front matter
doi:10.1016/j.hoc.2008.01.006

rather it represents the portals into the many dimensions of cancer survivorship and advocacy.

CANCER ADVOCACY ORGANIZATIONS: GENERAL

This list includes selected advocacy organizations that contain cancer-related information for patients who have any type of cancer. Survivorship and post-treatment resources are highlighted.

American Cancer Society (http://www.cancer.org)
>Cancer Survivors Network—http://www.acscsn.org
>>Along with standard information about resources, specific diseases, and treatments, the Cancer Survivors Network discusses posttreatment issues, offers chat rooms, and describes healthy lifestyle choices.
>Cancer Action Network—http://www.acscan.org
>>A nonprofit, nonpartisan sister advocacy organization of the American Cancer Society, the ACS CAN is dedicated to eliminating cancer as a major public health problem through voter education and issue-targeted campaigns to influence candidates and lawmakers to support relevant legislation and policies.

American Institute for Cancer Research (http://www.aicr.org)
Although diet and cancer prevention are the focus for the American Institute for Cancer Research, the Web site has a general category/link for cancer survivors. Resources include diet and exercise tips, recipes, support organizations, reading resources, and conferences. There is also access to free nutrition brochures along with books for purchase, including those by nutritionist and cancer survivor Diana Dyers.

American Society of Clinical Oncology (http://www.asco.org)
This Web site is for the more than 25,000 oncology practitioners who belong to the American Society of Clinical Oncology (ASCO) and represent all disciplines in oncology. Guidelines for long-term follow-up care are in development, and treatment summaries for breast and colorectal cancers are already available. The Web site audience includes patients and survivors.

>People Living With Cancer
>>Information for patients, including a section on survivorship. Survivors can find links to late effects, rehabilitation, childhood cancer survivorship, resources, and treatment summaries (printable).

Association of Cancer Online Resources (http://www.acor.org)
>Long-term Survivors Listserv—http://www.LT-Survivors@listserv.acor.org
>>More than 150 online discussion lists representing specific cancers and related disorders provide support, information, and community. The long-term survivors list offers opportunities to connect with others for discussions surrounding posttreatment issues. Information about clinics and resources are shared online and archived for later access. All lists are monitored.

Intercultural Cancer Council (http://iccnetwork.org)
The Intercultural Cancer Council focuses on cancer-related issues for ethnic minorities and medically underserved populations in the United States and its associated territories. Its survivor link takes you directly to resources on the Centers for Disease Control and Prevention Web site.

Lance Armstrong Foundation (http://www.livestrong.org)
The Lance Armstrong Foundation (LAF) provides grants for community programs, survivorship centers of excellence, and research efforts. It also offers information, support, and resources to patients, survivors, family members, and caregivers.

> The LIVESTRONG Survivorship Notebook can be ordered free of charge to help organize and manage information related to the cancer experience. Also, worksheets and information on special topics can be downloaded to personalize the notebook.
> Advocacy initiatives include LiveStrong Day and making cancer a national priority.

National Cancer Institute (http://www.cancer.gov)
Although information about survivorship does not appear on the main page of this Web site, if the word "survivorship" is typed, several references emerge. These include the following:

> Office of Cancer Survivorship—http://survivorship.cancer.gov
>   Provides grants for quality-of-life and long-term survivor research.
> Facing Forward: Ways You Can Make a Difference
> Facing Forward: Life After Cancer Treatment
> Facing Forward: When Someone You Love Has Completed Treatment
> Follow-up After Cancer Treatment: Questions and Answers

CancerCare (http://www.cancercare.org)
CancerCare is a national nonprofit organization whose mission is to provide free professional help to people who have all types of cancer through counseling, education, information and referral, and direct financial assistance.

> Annual Survivorship Series: Living With, Through, and Beyond Cancer. These telephone education workshops can be accessed in real time or as archived sessions.

National Coalition for Cancer Survivorship (http://www.canceradvocacy.org)
The National Coalition for Cancer Survivorship (NCCS) endorses evidence-based advocacy to implement systematic changes at the federal level in how the nation researches, regulates, finances, and delivers quality cancer care.

> NCCS organizes Cancer Advocacy Now!, a legislative advocacy network that engages constituents across the country in federal cancer-related issues.
> The NCCS award-winning Cancer Survival Toolbox is a set of skill-building CDs that is available free of charge in both English and Spanish. A Mandarin

translation is available in written format only. Living Beyond Cancer is module #10 in the series, and focuses on posttreatment issues.

National Comprehensive Cancer Network (http://www.nccn.org)

The National Comprehensive Cancer Network is an alliance of leading cancer centers that acts as an authoritative source of information for informed decision making about cancer care. It develops, updates, and disseminates a complete library of clinical practice guidelines. Some of the individual cancer-specific guidelines include information about long-term follow-up. This site also has an extensive list of cancer resource links for patients that includes sites related to research, cancer site–specific cancer organizations, and clinical trial groups.

Oncology Nursing Society (http://www.ons.org)

As the largest oncology organization in the world, the main focus of this nursing organization is the care of patients receiving treatment of cancer. Although much of the research in the field of survivorship has been done by oncology nurse researchers, there is little information on this site specifically for cancer survivors. First click on Patient Education, then link to Patient Support. Survivorship is included in this listing, and a limited list of resources can then be found.

> Cancer Symptoms.org—http://www.cancersymptoms.org
> This helpful Web site has been designed by ONS for patients and caregivers and provides information about 10 major symptoms frequently experienced during cancer treatment. These include anorexia, cognitive dysfunction, depression, dyspnea, fatigue, hormonal disturbances, neutropenia, pain, peripheral neuropathy, and sexual dysfunction. This site is useful for patients during and after treatment.

CHILDHOOD, ADOLESCENT, AND YOUNG ADULT ISSUES

These links offer a wide array of information about resources, treatments, research, and support for survivors of childhood cancer.

> Candlelighters—http://www.candlelighters.org
> Children's Oncology Group—http://www.childrensoncologygroup.org
> National Childhood Cancer Foundation—http://www.curesearch.org

Information available to survivors diagnosed with cancer as adolescents or young adults is outlined below.

American Society for Reproductive Medicine (http://www.asrm.org)

The ASRM is a nationally and internationally recognized leader for its provision of multidisciplinary information, education, advocacy, and standards in reproductive medicine. The Web site has links to general patient resources, particularly regarding fertility issues.

American Urological Association (http://www.auanet.org)

The American Urological Association provides courses in sexual medicine, including dysfunction in male and female cancer survivors.

Fertile Hope (http://www.fertilehope.org)

Fertile Hope is a national nonprofit organization dedicated to providing reproductive information, support, and hope to cancer patients whose medical treatments may result in infertility. Not only does this site offer a wealth of general information and resources but it also offers a way to calculate one's risk for infertility depending on disease and treatment. It was created by a young cancer survivor.

I'm Too Young For This (http://imtooyoungforthis.org)

The I'm Too Young For This (i[2]y!) Cancer Foundation is a leading survivor-led advocacy group working on behalf of survivors and caregivers younger than 40 years of age. This somewhat irreverent Web site provides resources, peer support, and social networks to young adults who have cancer. The site has an extensive list of organizations that offer exclusive support to young adults, including financial assistance, chat rooms, camps and retreats, blogs, literature, and advocacy tools.

> The Stupid Cancer Show http://imtooyoungforthis.org/stupidcancershow/ Hosted by i[2]y Founder, Matthew Zachary, The Stupid Cancer Show is a pioneering new interactive talk radio broadcast that gives voice to more than 1 million young adults affected by cancer.

Planet Cancer (http://planetcancer.com)

Planet Cancer is an international network of young adults, ready and willing to help each other through what may well be the most difficult experience of their lives. The underlying motivational tenet is that once you face cancer, there is little that you cannot do. The site is filled with resources designed to appeal to young adults who have cancer, including movies, videos, books, music, and various Top 10 lists.

Pregnant with Cancer Network (http://www.pregnantwithcancer.org)

This Web site connects women who are pregnant during their cancer experience. The site even attempts to match women who have the same type of cancer. It includes resource lists and newsletters.

Young Survival Coalition (http://www.youngsurvival.org)

The Young Survival Coalition is an international organization dedicated to the concerns and issues that are unique to young women who have breast cancer, especially those who are aged 40 years and younger. The site has an expansive resource list, including one for special populations and those living with metastatic disease. The link to survivorship falls under Wellness and Moving Forward. It is filled with information about nutrition and exercise, beauty and body image, retreats and adventures, spirituality and religion, moving forward and becoming a parent, getting involved, and advocacy.

Young Cancer Spouses (http://www.youngcancerspouses.com)

The following comes from the vision statement of this organization: "The needs of young spouses of cancer patients often go unrecognized and unappreciated. The emotional and logistical issues that a young spouse of a cancer patient faces are vastly different from spouses of older cancer patients that dominated oncology units and support groups. General family support groups are likewise inadequate at addressing the needs of a young cancer spouse" [1]. Resources include tips about caring for the patient and caregiver, relationships, and financial matters.

CANCER TREATMENT SUMMARIES
Since the publication of the Institute of Medicine's report, *From Cancer Patient to Cancer Survivor: Lost in Transition*, the oncology community has created various formats for treatment summaries and care plans [2].

American Society of Clinical Oncology (http://www.asco.org)
ASCO has Cancer Treatment Summaries, Survivorship Care Plans, and Follow-up Care currently available for breast and colorectal cancers. The formats can be downloaded. Work continues on plans and follow-up care for other types of cancer.

Oncolink: Oncolife Survivorship Care Plan (http://www.oncolink.org/oncolife)
The Abramson Cancer Center of the University of Pennsylvania developed OncoLink, the Web's first cancer resource. This site provides all categories of resources, including a survivorship link, and the OncoLife Survivorship Care Plan. In this latter plan, survivors can enter their treatment information and receive an individualized, basic care plan that can then be reviewed with one's own health care team. It is meant to serve as a springboard for in-depth discussion and personal interpretation with one's physician or oncology provider.

ADULT RETREATS AND CAMPS
Children and adolescents have been using camps and retreats to support healing and recovery from cancer for quite some time. Adults have recently discovered the healing potential of this type of informal support, and programs have multiplied nationwide, with several highlighted here.

Survivors' Retreat (http://www.survivorsretreat.com)
This general Web site was created by a cancer survivor who collects information about retreats, spa opportunities, workshops, and conferences. The focus is on women's programs, but many include family members. Programs can be filtered by theme (healing, activities, renewal); by type of participants (specific cancer, all cancers, young adults, and so forth); by location, or by cost.

    Adirondack Arts and Healing Retreat—Camp Sagamore—http://sagamore.org
    American Cancer Society (varies by state)—http://www.cancer.org
    Betty J. Borry Breast Cancer Retreats (New Hampshire)—http://bjbbreastcan cerretreats.org
    Bluebird Cancer Retreats (Michigan)—http://bluebirdmi.org

BlueBonnet Retreat—Harris Methodist Hospital Foundation (Texas)—http://www.texashealth.org/hospitals/def

Breast Cancer Recovery—The Women's Wilderness Institute (Colorado)—http://www.womenswilderness.org/womens_p

Camp Bravehearts (New York, Pennsylvania)—http://braveheartscamp.org

Camp Good Days (New York)—http://campgooddays.org

Camp Mak-a-Dream (Montana)—http://www.campdream.org

Cancer as a Turning Point (Connecticut)—http://cancerasaturningpoint.org

Cancer Care Resources (Oregon)—http://cancercareresources.org

CancerFit Walking Program (Arizona)—http://www.wellbeyond.com

Canyon Ranch—Dream Street Foundation (Arizona)—http://www.DreamStreetFoundation.org

Casting for Recovery (Vermont)—http://www.castingforrecovery.org

Commonweal Cancer Help Program (CCHP) (Calif)—http://commonweal.org

Cordelia Knott Center for Wellness (Southern California)—http://ckwellnesscenter.org

Creative Healing Retreat—Enhancement, Inc. (California)—http://enhancementinc.org

Family Cancer Retreat—Cancer Services of New Mexico—http://cancerservicesnm.org

F. Holland Day Center for Healing (Maine)—http://fhollanddaycenter.org

First Descents (Colorado, Montana)—http://firstdescents.org

From Surviving to Thriving—The Mary Macguire Foundation (Ohio, Kentucky)—http://marymaguirefoundation.org

Harmony Hill Retreat Center (Washington)—http://harmonyhill.org

Healing Odyssey (California)—http://healingodyssey.org

Healing with Horses—Life Management, Inc. (North Carolina)—http://lifemanagementinc.org

Infinite Boundaries Retreats (Wisconsin)—http://bcrf.org

Insights for Living Beyond Cancer at the Mind and Body Wellness Center (Pennsylvania)—http://ecap-online.org/retreat.htm

Journey Through Cancer & The Seven Levels of Healing (Texas, New York)—http://www.geffenvisions.com

KoKoLuLu Cancer Retreats (Hawaii)—http://www.cancer-retreats.org

Libby Ross Foundation (New York City)—http://thelibbyrossfoundation.com

Life Beyond Cancer (Arizona)—http://www.lifebeyondcancer.com

Mak-A-Dream Ovarian Cancer Retreat (Montana)—http://campdream.org

Mending in the Mountains (Montana)—http://center4support.org

Mending Under the Moon (N. California)—http://MarinCancerInstitute.org

Next Step (Massachusetts, Connecticut)—http://nextstepnet.org

Planet Cancer (Texas)—http://www.planetcancer.org

Reel Recovery (Massachusetts)—http://www.reelrecovery.org

Reeling and Healing Midwest (Michigan and Illinois)—http://www.reelingandhealingmidwest.org

Smith Farm Center for the Healing Arts (Maryland)—http://smithfarm.com

Stepping Stone Spa and Wellness Center (Vermont)—http://steppingstonewellnesscenter.com

Stowe Weekend of Hope (Vermont)—http://stowehope.org

Sunstone Healing Center (Arizona)—http://sunstonehealing.org

Young Adult Cancer Survivor Retreat (Tennessee)—http://www.minnie
pearl.org

Women Beyond Cancer (Missouri, South Carolina, Utah)—http://women
beyondcancer.org

SURVIVORSHIP PUBLICATIONS AND EDUCATIONAL TOOLS

Cancer Survival Toolbox (http://www.cancersurvivaltoolbox.org)

This educational tool is offered free of charge from the National Coalition for
Cancer Survivorship (see earlier section in this article). The toolbox is available
in CD format or can be accessed online in English and Spanish. This resource
includes skill-building techniques along with special topics for older people,
caregivers, the uninsured, and long-term survivors. New modules will include
self-navigation and end-of-life issues.

CURE: Cancer Updates, Research, & Education
(http://www.curetoday.com)

CURE is a magazine developed for individuals coping with cancer and
hematologic diseases. CURE provides scientific information in an easy-to-
understand format on topics related to diagnosis and treatment of cancer. It
is provided to clinics and individuals free of charge.

Facing Forward Series (http://www.cancer.gov)

Facing Forward: Ways You Can Make a Difference in Cancer
Facing Forward: Life After Cancer Treatment
Facing Forward: When Someone You Love Has Completed Treatment

This information is available at no cost by calling 1-800-4-CANCER (1-800-
422-6237) or online at http://www.cancer.gov.

Heal: Living Well after Cancer (http://www.healtoday.com)

From the publishers of CURE magazine, Heal explores the area of life after
cancer or when initial treatment ends. It includes the many dimensions of
survivorship and long-term survival.

Live Strong Educational Tools and Survivorship Notebook
(http://www.livestrong.org)

An educational program of the LAF, Live Strong is a resource created to
educate survivors and their friends, families, and caregivers about cancer survivorship. From the moment cancer survivorship begins on the first day of
diagnosis, this site provides the information and tools needed to "live
strong."

OTHER ADVOCACY ORGANIZATIONS

Center for Patient Advocacy (http://www.patientadvocate.org)

The Center for Patient Advocacy advocates for patient rights and aids cancer
patients in navigating managed health care by way of its Web site, free publications, quarterly newsletter, and telephone hotline.

Patient Access Network Foundation (http://www.patientaccessnetwork.org)
The Patient Access Network Foundation is dedicated to supporting the needs of patients who cannot access needed treatments because of insufficient monetary resources.

Patient Advocate Foundation (http://www.patientadvocate.org)
The Patient Advocate Foundation is a national nonprofit organization that serves as an active liaison between the patient and his or her insurer, employer, or creditors to resolve insurance, job retention, or debt crisis matters relative to a cancer diagnosis. Access is provided to case managers, doctors, and legal support.

COMMENT

Advocacy efforts range from helping another cancer survivor during one-on-one informal settings to the creation of nonprofit organizations. We can choose to advocate for ourselves and our family members for access to quality cancer care or to advocate for general resources within our community. Some of us are able to raise funds for cancer research by participating in organized walks or runs. Others can serve as teachers to fellow survivors, caregivers, and health care providers. We may also offer support through veteran–rookie survivor mentoring relationships, by serving as watchdogs within business and government agencies, by playing a role as consumer advocates for research trials, or by becoming involved in public policy and national system changes. No matter what our primary focus, there is always an opportunity to make a difference. The listings of cancer advocacy organizations, programs, and educational materials in this article provide only a sampling of what is available to the general public and serve as a valuable starting point to anyone affected by cancer.

References

[1] Available at: http://www.youngcancerspouses.com/about/about_mission.html.
[2] Institute of Medicine. In: Hewitt M, Greenfield S, Stovall E, editors. From Cancer patient to cancer survivor: lost in transition. Washington, DC: The National Academies Press; 2006. Available at: http://www.nap.edu.

Cancer Survivorship: Facing Forward

Lois B. Travis, MD, ScD[a],*, Joachim Yahalom, MD[b]

[a]Division of Cancer Epidemiology and Genetics, National Cancer Institute, Department of Health and Human Services, National Institutes of Health, Bethesda, MD, USA
[b]Department of Radiation Oncology, Memorial Sloan-Kettering Cancer Center, 1275 York Avenue, New York, NY 10021, USA

B ased on cancer incidence rates in 2002 to 2004, it is estimated that 40.9% of men and women born today in the United States will be diagnosed with some type of cancer [1]. An even larger number of people know someone who has survived cancer, underscoring the impact of cancer on the public. The ranks of cancer survivors numbered 10.7 million in 2004, representing 3.5% of the United States population [1]. Since the institution of the National Cancer Act in 1971, the number of cancer survivors in the United States has tripled, and is growing by 2% each year [2]. The burgeoning number of patients reflects improvements throughout the cancer continuum, including early detection, supportive care, and therapeutic approaches. Among all cancer patients, the 5-year relative survival rate is now 64.9% [1]. Thus, a growing constituency lives among us to advocate for issues related to cancer survivorship.

CANCER SURVIVORSHIP: THE PAST

In 1986, the National Coalition for Cancer Survivorship was founded [3]. Despite the small number of charter members (only 23), NCCS gave birth to an era in which a new term was added to the language of oncology, one that heightened the importance of looking past the time beyond cancer treatment to a patient's future. In 1996, the National Cancer Institute (NCI) established the Office of Cancer Survivorship (OCS) [4], with a mission to improve the length and quality of life of all people diagnosed with cancer. OCS accomplishes its goals through activities in several areas: the provision of research support, the training of researchers and clinicians dedicated to studying and caring for cancer survivors, and the development of educational materials and outreach programs. The domains of cancer survivorship research, as articulated by Aziz and Rowland of OCS [5], include descriptive and analytic research, intervention research, follow-up care and surveillance, family and caregiver issues, economic impact, health disparities, and instrument development. This prioritization of cancer survivorship by the NCI and the founding

*Corresponding author. 1275 East First Avenue, #159, New York, NY 10065.
E-mail address: travis1122@optonline.net (L.B. Travis).

0889-8588/08/$ – see front matter
doi:10.1016/j.hoc.2008.01.009

of the OCS have been mirrored in a tripling of PubMed citations related to adult cancer survivorship research between 1992 and 2004 (from 132 to 374 publications) [6]. Nonetheless, these numbers remain miniscule compared with the number of citations for adult cancer treatment research in 1992 and 2004 (11,298 and 23,736, respectively). Discrepancies reflect the recent establishment of this discipline, the relatively modest levels of research support, and the need for extended periods of follow-up [6]. Nonetheless, progress continues.

In November 2004, the NCI sponsored a workshop, the major objective of which was to provide perspective on the research agenda, design considerations, and infrastructure needed to understand the underlying genetic mechanisms of late neoplastic effects in cancer survivors and thus to facilitate the development of evidence-based long-term management and intervention strategies. The workshop proceedings were published as a Commentary in the first issue of 2006 of the *Journal of the National Cancer Institute* [7]. Although the focus of the workshop was second primary cancers, participants emphasized that most of the infrastructural and design approaches that supported research in this area also provided a sound basis for the study of other important physiologic late effects and psychosocial concerns in cancer survivors.

In 2006 the American Society for Clinical Oncology (ASCO) introduced a "Patient Care and Survivor Care" track to its annual meeting. In November of the same year ASCO devoted an issue of *Journal of Clinical Oncology* to survivorship concerns. In addition to these efforts, recent seminal publications by the Institute of Medicine (IOM) [6,8], the President's Cancer Panel [9,10], and a joint report from the Centers for Disease Control and Prevention and the Lance Armstrong Foundation [11] have drawn additional attention to the growing field of survivorship research and care.

CANCER SURVIVORSHIP: PRESENT CHALLENGES AND FUTURE OPPORTUNITIES

The critical question is, where do we go from here? In the IOM Report [6], one chapter was devoted to future challenges in survivorship research, with recommendations summarized in Box 1. Because much of this issue is devoted to concerns surrounding physiologic late sequelae in cancer survivors, in this article we highlight opportunities for research in these areas. Although the research community has made notable advances in delineating treatment-associated risks for late effects, particularly second primary cancers, the identification of patient subgroups that might be at heightened susceptibility to developing various adverse sequelae has not been systematically addressed. Although there is little information on the molecular underpinnings of genetic susceptibility to the development of late effects in the growing population of cancer survivors, the meticulous measurement and documentation of potentially carcinogenic treatments (chemotherapy and radiotherapy) serve as a strong basis for the study of gene–environment and gene–gene interactions. In addition, an important opportunity exists to investigate the role of effect modifiers of treatment effects

Box 1: Institute of Medicine and National Research Council report: future areas for cancer survivorship research

Mechanisms of late effects experienced by cancer survivors

How to identify and intervene to alleviate symptoms and improve function

The prevalence and risk of late effects

The cost effectiveness of alternative models of survivorship care and community-based psychosocial services

    Post-treatment surveillance strategies and interventions

    Survivors' and caregivers' attitudes and preferences regarding outcomes and survivorship care

    Needs of racial/ethnic groups, residents of rural areas, and other potentially underserved groups

    Supportive care and rehabilitation programs

Interventions to improve quality of life

    Family and caregiver needs and access to supportive services

    Mechanisms to reduce financial burdens of survivorship care

    Employer programs to meet return-to-work needs

    Approaches to improve health insurance coverage

    Legal protections afforded cancer survivors through the Americans with Disabilities Act, Family and Medical Leave Act, HIPAA, and other laws

Survivorship research methods

    Barriers to participation

    Impact of HIPAA

    Methods to overcome challenges of survivorship research (eg, methods to adjust for bias introduced by nonparticipation, methods to minimize loss to follow-up)

Abbreviation: HIPPA, Health Insurance Portability and Accountability Act.
Adapted from Hewitt M, Greenfield S, Stovall E. From cancer patient to cancer survivor: lost in transition. Washington, DC: National Academies Press; 2005. p.468; with permission.

(eg, tobacco use) [12]. To date, however, there has been no concerted effort to provide future research direction in this complex area. Because molecular markers to gauge patient prognosis and predict tumor response to treatment are under investigation [13–15], it seems timely that attempts to customize therapy could also incorporate factors that might predict the susceptibility of patients to acute and chronic toxicity. Prospective identification of patients genetically susceptible to the late complications of cancer treatment [16] could result in opportunities to individualize therapy to maximize therapeutic benefit and to minimize serious late toxicity [17]. Further perspective on the research agenda, design considerations, and infrastructure needed to understand the underlying genetic mechanisms of late neoplastic effects in cancer survivors and thus to facilitate the development of evidence-based long-term management and intervention strategies was considered during the November 2004 NCI workshop and reviewed in detail elsewhere [7]. In Box 2, the recommendations of this group are summarized. Note that the recommendations included provisions for infrastructure development, including support for the collection and storage of biospecimens, and the development of new technology, bioinformatics, and biomarkers.

As did participants at the NCI-convened workshop [7], the IOM Report [6] underscored the need to study large numbers of patients who survive their cancers for many years to detect unusual late effects. Still larger numbers are needed to effectively study gene–environment interactions. As pointed out by participants at the 2004 NCI-sponsored workshop [7], the IOM report reiterated that one mechanism to accrue large numbers of cancer survivors who represent the diversity of the United States population is to conduct multi-institutional collaborative research [6]. One such large program (CONCURED) is now being organized by investigators at the Wilmot Cancer Center, Rochester, New York [18], with a goal of the inclusion of minority and underserved populations. At the most recent meeting of this group of investigators (May 2007), more than 20 major institutions were represented in a voluntary effort to enroll patients onto common survivorship protocols. Importantly, the topic of prospectively establishing biobanks was discussed. It is highly likely that the CONCURED effort, when fully mature, will have sufficient statistical power to address the role of gene–environment interactions in the production of late effects. Analytic studies of cancer survivors thus now enter the realm of big science, a research approach recently described by Hoover [19]. A particularly pragmatic issue that researchers who contribute to large consortia must begin to consider is how to ensure that junior investigators receive appropriate recognition for their efforts [20].

Until the results of analytic research undertaken in large survivorship cohorts are available, how do we care for cancer survivors? It is clear that scientific progress over the last few decades has made it possible to identify those treatment regimens that are associated with high risks for late effects. Although individual susceptibility factors may remain largely unknown, selected groups of patients can still be chosen for close monitoring, and consensus-based guidelines can be issued. One excellent model for this latter approach is the comprehensive guidelines created by the Children's Oncology Group for the management of late effects; these were developed through consensus procedures among panels of experts [21]. Because the treatments itemized in the guidelines have also been used to treat cancer in adults, this set of recommendations serves as one starting point for the follow-up of adult cancer survivors until evidence-based guidelines have been independently generated. Recently, ASCO proposed consensus-based guidelines for the follow-up of cardiac and pulmonary late effects in cancer survivors [22]. Other consensus-based recommendations from respected sources, such as the National Comprehensive Cancer Network [23], which include guidelines for patient follow-up, also provide needed direction for health care providers.

Box 2: National Cancer Institute–sponsored workshop: recommendations for future research

Develop research infrastructure for studies of cancer survivorship

Institute a systematic, national approach to develop research infrastructure for studies of genetic modifiers of late effects of cancer treatment, including second malignancies.

Provide for rigorous ascertainment of multiple primary cancers with clinical annotation, detailed treatment data, and biospecimen collection.

Establish multicenter cohorts of cancer survivors, with recruitment of transdisciplinary research teams dedicated to researching the late effects of therapy.

Expand the capacity of National Cancer Institute cooperative groups to ascertain and study long-term outcomes in clinical trial populations, in support of survivorship research.

Create a coordinated system for biospecimen collection

Standardize biospecimen collection, laboratory procedures, and documentation for blood and other DNA sources, normal tissue from target organs, and tumor tissue.

Develop a centralized biospecimen repository or a tracking system ("virtual repository") to permit sample retrieval from multiple storage centers. Institute mechanisms for scientific review of specimen use and administrative procedures for specimen control.

Support methodologic research to enhance the quality and lower the cost of biospecimen collection, processing, storage, and distribution.

Promote the development of new technology, bioinformatics, and biomarkers

Identify new technologies for the analysis of germline and somatic genetic alterations to determine their contributions to second cancer risk.

Reduce the amount of tissue and DNA needed for various assays, with standardization of protocols for whole genome amplification.

Develop molecular profiles of tumors that incorporate analyses of etiologic pathways and therapeutic targets related to second cancers and other late outcomes.

Support the development of new epidemiologic methods

Develop efficient epidemiologic study designs to investigate the role of genetic susceptibility to multiple primary cancers, including genetic modifiers of risk associated with treatment effects or other etiologic factors.

Develop optimal approaches for selection of controls for case-control studies in which treatment and genetic susceptibility play important roles.

Include a biospecimen component in all study designs.

Develop evidence-based clinical practice guidelines

Implement pilot studies of interventions to prevent second cancers within genetically defined, high-risk groups of patients.

Integrate smoking cessation programs into research designs.

Support research to provide evidence-based follow-up care for cancer survivors.

Adapted from Travis LB, Rabkin CS, Brown LM, et al. Cancer survivorship-genetic susceptibility and second primary cancers: research strategies and recommendations. J Natl Cancer Inst 2006;98(1):15–25; with permission.

For now, cancer survivors should also be encouraged to adopt practices that are consistent with a healthy lifestyle, including smoking cessation; to seek medical consultation for any persistent changes in health status; and, as a starting point, to follow screening guidelines applicable to the general population [24]. Where consensus-based guidelines for specific patient populations and treatment exposures have been developed, these should also be implemented. Even though cancer therapy represents a double-edged sword, many new treatments and management strategies resulted in sizable improvements in patient survival, and have ushered in an era of the "problem of success." The benefits associated with many cancer treatments greatly exceed the risk for developing adverse effects, although risk-adapted therapy should now be implemented whenever possible. Moreover, the evolving era of targeted therapy and personalized medicine will provide an opportunity to tailor treatment to the patient, taking into account tumor characteristics, the patient's underlying genetic profile, the existence of comorbidities, and the patient's susceptibility to the late complications of specific treatments.

It should always be kept in mind that the adverse effects of cancer and its treatment may not necessarily be attributable to prior therapy, but also reflect the effect of shared etiologic factors, environmental exposures, host characteristics, patient comorbidities, underlying hepatic and renal function, lifestyle factors, and combinations of influences, including gene–environment and gene–gene interactions [25]. Research undertaken in large well-constructed cohorts of survivors should be able to clarify the roles of these various influences on the risk for late effects, identify genetically susceptible populations, and also provide the basis for evidence-based prevention and intervention efforts [7].

Acknowledgments

We thank Ms. Janice Chau for editorial support.

References

[1] Ries L, Melbert D, Krapcho M, et al. SEER Cancer Statistics Review, 1975–2004. Bethesda (MD): National Cancer Institute; 2007.

[2] Cancer survivors: living longer, and now, better [editorial]. Lancet 2004;364(9452): 2153–4.

[3] Hoffman B. A cancer survivor's almanac: charting your journey. 3rd edition. Hoboken (NJ): John Wiley & Sons Inc.; 2004.

[4] Institute NC. National Cancer Institute: cancer survivorship research. Available at: http://dccps.nci.nih.gov/ocs/.

[5] Aziz NM, Rowland JH. Trends and advances in cancer survivorship research: challenge and opportunity. Semin Radiat Oncol 2003;13(3):248–66.

[6] Hewitt M, Greenfield S, Stovall E. From cancer patient to cancer survivor: lost in transition. Washington, DC: National Academies Press; 2005.

[7] Travis LB, Rabkin CS, Brown LM, et al. Cancer survivorship—genetic susceptibility and second primary cancers: research strategies and recommendations. J Natl Cancer Inst 2006;98(1):15–25.

[8] Hewitt M, Weiner S, Simone J. Childhood cancer survivorship: improving care and quality of life. Washington, DC: The National Academies Press; 2003.

[9] Services USDoHaH. Living beyond cancer: finding a new balance: President's Cancer Panel 2003/2004 Annual Report. Bethesda (MD) 2004.

[10] Services USDoHaH. Assessing progress: advancing change: President's Cancer Panel 2005/2006 Annual Report 2006.

[11] Prevention CfDCa. Centers for Disease Control and Prevention and the Lance Armstrong Foundation: A national action plan for cancer survivorship: advancing public health strategies. Atlanta (GA): 2004.

[12] Travis LB, Gospodarowicz M, Curtis RE, et al. Lung cancer following chemotherapy and radiotherapy for Hodgkin's disease. J Natl Cancer Inst 2002;94(3):182–92.

[13] Van't Veer LJ, Dai H, Van De Vijver MJ, et al. Gene expression profiling predicts clinical outcome of breast cancer. Nature 2002;415(6871):530–6.

[14] Ayers M, Symmans WF, Stec J, et al. Gene expression profiles predict complete pathologic response to neoadjuvant paclitaxel and fluorouracil, doxorubicin, and cyclophosphamide chemotherapy in breast cancer. J Clin Oncol 2004;22(12):2284–93.

[15] Paik S, Shak S, Tang G, et al. A multigene assay to predict recurrence of tamoxifen-treated, node-negative breast cancer. N Engl J Med 2004;351(27):2817–26.

[16] Khoury MJ, Yang Q, Gwinn M, et al. An epidemiologic assessment of genomic profiling for measuring susceptibility to common diseases and targeting interventions. Genet Med 2004;6(1):38–47.

[17] Bast RC Jr, Hortobagyi GN. Individualized care for patients with cancer—a work in progress. N Engl J Med 2004;351(27):2865–9.

[18] Travis LB. Defining the leading edge in research of adverse effects of cancer treatment. Semin Radiat Oncol, in press.

[19] Hoover RN. The evolution of epidemiologic research from cottage industry to "big" science. Epidemiology 2007;18(1):13–7.

[20] Ness RB. "Big" science and the little guy. Epidemiology 2007;18(1):9–12.

[21] Group CsO. Long-term follow-up guidelines for survivors of childhood and young adult cancers. Available at: http://www.survivorshipguidelines.org/.

[22] Carver JR, Shapiro CL, Ng A, et al. American Society of Clinical Oncology clinical evidence review on the ongoing care of adult cancer survivors: cardiac and pulmonary late effects. J Clin Oncol 2007;25(25):3991–4008.

[23] Network NCC. Welcome to the NCCN clinical practice in oncology. Available at: http://www.nccn.org/professionals/physician_gls/default.asp.

[24] Smith RA, Cokkinides V, Eyre HJ. American Cancer Society guidelines for the early detection of cancer, 2004. CA Cancer J Clin 2004;54(1):41–52.

[25] Travis LB. Therapy-associated solid tumors. Acta Oncol 2002;41(4):323–33.

INDEX

A

Acquired somatic genetics, and cancer survivorship, 257–259

Acupuncture, for cancer survivors, 345

Adolescents, survivorship advocacy organizations and support systems, 358–360

Adult cancer survivors. *See* Survivors, cancer.

Advocacy, cancer survivorship organizations and support systems, **355–363**
    adult retreats and camps, 360–362
    cancer treatment summaries, 360
    childhood, adolescent, and young adult issues, 358–360
    general, 356–358
    others, 362–363
    survivorship publications and educational tools, 362

American Cancer Institute, 356

American Institute for Cancer Research, 356

American Society for Reproductive Medicine, 358

American Society of Clinical Oncology, 356

American Urological Association, 358

Anthracyclines, cardiac toxicity related to cancer therapy with, 305–307

Association of Cancer Online Resources, 356

B

Behavior change, in promoting healthy lifestyle for cancer survivors, 334–336

Botanicals, for cancer survivors, 349–350

Breast cancer, fertility in young cancer survivors with, 294
    heart disease following radiation therapy for, 311–312
    screening for, in long-term survivors of Hodgkin's lymphoma, 233–234
    second primary malignancies after, 277–279
    sexuality in young cancer survivors with, 298–299

C

Camps, for adult cancer survivors, 360–362

CancerCare, 357

Cancers, second. *See* Second malignancies.

Carbohydrate intake, in healthy diet for cancer survivors, 329–331

Cardiovascular complications, long-term, of cancer therapy, **305–318**
    cardiac toxicity,
        anthracycline-related, 305–307
        taxanes-related, 307
        trastuzumab-related, 307–308
    pulmonary toxicity, late chemotherapy- or radiation-induced, 314–315
    radiation-induced, delayed
        pericarditis, 312–313
        myocardial dysfunction, 313
        valvular disease, 313–314
    radiation-related cardiovascular complications, 308–312
        coronary heart disease in Hodgkin's lymphoma patients, 308–311
        detection of coronary heart disease, 312
        heart disease in breast cancer patients, 311–312

Cardiovascular disease, in long-term follow-up of testicular cancer patients, 248–249
    screening and prevention in long-term survivors of Hodgkin's lymphoma, 236–238
        coronary artery disease, 237–238
        evaluation of symptoms, 238
        ventricular dysfunction, 237

Care planning, survivorship, for adult cancer survivors, **201–210**
    survivorship care plans, 203–206
        implementation of, 206–208
    teachable moments, 208–209

Note: Page numbers of article titles are in **boldface** type.

0889-8588/08/$ – see front matter
doi:10.1016/S0889-8588(08)00048-8